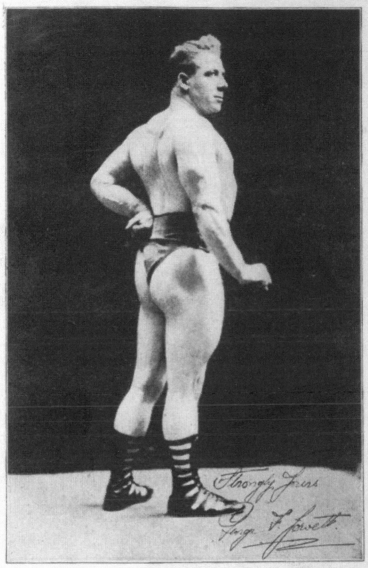

The author, George F. Jowett, whose career as an athlete, teacher, writer
and soldier of fortune, will always forcibly remain in the mind of strength
followers and body builders, as one of our greatest inspirations.

Key to Might and Muscle

By
GEORGE F. JOWETT

Founder and President of American Continental Weight
Lifters' Association. One of the World's Strongest Athletes

Originally Published in 1926

PUBLISHED BY O'Faolain Patriot LLC, Copyright 2011
info@PhysicalCultureBooks.com
Published in the United States of America

ISBN-13: 978-1466400870

ISBN-10: 1466400870

To Order More Copies Visit: Physical Culture Books.com

The information contained in this publication is for historical and educational purposes only and is not designed to and does not provide medical, nutritional, or health advice, diagnosis, or opinion for any health or individual problem. The material presented is not a substitute for medical or other professional health services from a qualified health care provider who is familiar with the unique facts of the individual, and should not be used in place of a visit, call, consultation, or advice of a physician or other healthcare provider. Individuals should always consult a qualified health care provider about any health concern and prior to undertaking any new treatment. The publisher assumes no responsibility and specifically disclaims all liability for any consequence relating directly or indirectly to any action or inaction that a reader takes based on any information contained herein.

Be advised that no one should undertake exercises in the nature of those addressed in this book without prior consultation with a physician. Nor does the publisher make any representations concerning whether any of the exercises or suggestions provided by the trainers or physical fitness specialists featured in this book would be effective or appropriate for the reader's needs or expectations. The publisher expressly disclaims any and all responsibility and/or liabilities that might result from the uninformed or misinformed application of the techniques identified herein as well as for any unsupervised physical fitness training.

Finally, the publisher disclaims any and all liabilities arising from the use of any equipment featured in this book and makes no representations as to the utility, safety, or adequacy of the equipment generally or with respect to any specific purpose.

TABLE OF CONTENTS

CHAPTER I
A FEW CHAPTERS FROM THE STORY OF MY LIFE

On a boiling hot summer day, rolling in a cloud of dust in the middle of the road, like two angry pups, were two young lads. They were eventually dragged apart, hardly recognizable on account of the mingled dirt, sweat and torn clothing. One was a much smaller chap than the other, and his face was very pale. In fact, he had just resumed school after leaving the hospital a few weeks before. This little chap had been in the hospital for eight years, more or less, through the result of an injury when only a six months old baby. Yet, he cried with mortification at being dragged away from his bigger opponent. He still wanted to lick the other chap even if it was a hopeless looking proposition. Somewhere in his mind was the belief that while the other chap got a belly full, he could at least get a mouthful. He did not think of the handicap of age, weight and strength. The poor little fair haired kid thought no one had the right to lick him, anyway. From that moment he harbored a thirst for revenge, and devoted all his spare time to exercises that would make him bigger and stronger. Somehow it dawned in his youthful mind that the right kind of exercise would provide the means best suited to enable him to lick his tormentor. This settled in his mind, he pitched into his training with a vengeance, studying the methods and devices that would grow muscle. He played at everything, wrestling with all the other boys he could get interested, and if he could not find enough kids interested, he started a fight. He was determined to get practice one way or another.

Well, the old proverb says that all comes to those who wait, and it came to little "curly head." He and his old tormentor met once more in a pitched battle, when curly licked the hide off the bigger boy.

The recital of this little story you have just read, is written here with a definite purpose in mind. As much as it is penned to gain your interest, the actual stimulus I want to create within you is determination, to inspire you to achieve, succeed. You must resolve within your heart and feel with a fixed determination that "what this man has done, so can I do."

This little story you have just read is taken from an article that was written about my life and published in the columns of a sports magazine. I was told by the editor that the story inspired many young fellows with that "do or die" disposition which has never failed to bring success to the aspirant. It made me very happy, for if there is any one thing in which I am sincere, it is the desire to help others secure the fullness of health, strength and manliness.

I have often thought that I never saw anything written about myself in as few words that portrayed my life battle like that true little story. It has a strong appeal to me, because every line, yes, every word throbs with a heartache, a joy, a longing to be, and back of it all, a determination to be some day a stronger man than the average. I want to inspire you with the same message of salvation and physical redemption, so that you will set your lips more tightly and step out with a fearless tread.

My early illness is something upon which I have seldom touched, because I am aware of the fact that such a claim was once a popular method of advertising, and I naturally resented any criticism that might have inferred that I was "just another." Many have asked me if my parents were strong, and truthfully I replied that they were very healthy people. When I was only six months of age, my mother let me fall from her lap in an effort to save my sister from being severely scalded. Unfortunately—or was it fortunately—I was the victim, and when they picked me up, I was bleeding.

In the fall I had injured my abdomen upon one of the iron ornaments that decorate open fireplaces. From then on it was a battle for life. Being so young nothing had matured, and certain internal organs were crippled and continued to remain in that injured condition. Nothing helped me. My life was a perpetual round of visits to physicians who did the best they could. As I grew in bodily size, my condition became more serious. Operation after operation was suggested, and I survived three. To this day, my memory visualizes the agonies of a bed of pain. I laid as though crucified with my hands, head and feet strapped down, and a cage over my body so that no clothing could touch my tortured flesh. I survived my last operation at the age of eight, and I can well remember how the tears filled my mother's eyes, as the doctor told her that nothing more could be done for me, and it was only a matter of time. Mother must realize that it was impossible for me to ever attain the age of fifteen. How this prediction failed of fulfillment is told in the fact that at the age of fifteen I commenced my professional athletic career, and two years before that I had won gymnastic honors. From then on it was a march over obstacles, even though I knew my path was still to be beset with many disappointments. I knew the answer. There remained no riddle in the sands for me. I knew that exercise was the great re-builder, and with my feet firmly set on the first step I began the climb. The fact that I knew my very life was at stake was the fundamental reason which led me so deeply into the field of physical research and investigation. Day by day I accumulated a practical knowledge that laid the foundation for my teachings and that knowledge I have placed before the health-seeking public for years now. In this volume, the reader will find every subject clarified in an earnest endeavor that he may also succeed.

The one great impression I want to create in your mind is the indelible fact that you are reading the results of the investigations of one who commenced life probably in a worse state than many, and therefore had to expend great efforts to win a better built body. This being the case, you will realize that I know what obstacles you have to meet, and how to sympathize with you in your bitter hours. Besides that I want to inject into you some of the inspiration that I had and still retain, the kind that positively refuses to back down. Make your inspiration, and you will then be an inspiration to others.

You know it is all in the way you handle yourself and whether you are game enough to secure the fullness of life.

Continuing with our heart to heart talk, let me explain to you how inspiration works with me. For example I am going to take you back a few years to my early days when I was just launching out as an athlete, and at the same time had been following the trails of the wanderlust for a period of years. I arrived in Rotterdam, Holland, where I starred under that famous Dutch athlete, Dirk Van der Berg, and in my spare moments I made various pilgrimages to the shrines of the great emancipators of liberty and thought. I visited the place where the great Russian leader, Peter the Great, served as a ship apprentice for the benefit of his country, and also the little garret where Erasmus, one of the early stars of the reformation, struggled with poverty and high ideals. The home of the DeWitts, the studio of Rubens, and the places that were haunted once by the Puritan Fathers, who after their journey from England waited and waited and waited around the quays for the ships that were to carry them to the land of promise.

Somehow those great men seemed to have left some of their greatness behind in those hallowed places to inspire hungry souls like mine, which were battling to achieve a life ambition. I would return to my companions saturated with renewed inspiration, and my impressive recitals, or ravings, would hold them enthralled as I retold the story of the great lives whose haunts I had daily visited.

They would actually scratch their heads and tell me that they never knew there were such places in Rotterdam and Amsterdam; and they had been around these places for many years.

The moral to this can be told in just a few words. The majority of those people were drones. Heedlessly they allowed inspired lessons that were right within their sight to pass by, like bread upon the waters. Many health seekers are the same. Only far away pastures seem green. To me those sights were sermons of flaming fire, that created within me an absorbing determination to live, to succeed, and not to die young. Back again, I would plunge into my studies of exercise, with a resolution that never recognized the word No.

When trials were hard to bear, I would think of the great men who had succeeded, and visualize how much harder their lot had been than mine. It was like wine to a drooping man.

It was at this time that the famous building at the Hague was completed; set up by Andrew Carnegie, a highly successful common man, for the diplomats of the world to meet in and establish a broader principle of right ruling rather than might. I journeyed with some comrades on bicycles to view this mass of stone, little thinking that within ten years the world would be deciding the questions asked by the donor of this monument with a sacrifice of many thousands of lives.

Years afterwards, when I stripped in the recruiting office in Ottawa, Canada, to enlist as a soldier to fight for that great principle, the examining physician, a man who had examined thousands upon thousands of specimens of manhood, stood back with an amazed look on his face as I stepped in line before him, and exclaimed, "My God, what a man."

Although I had won my battles years before this incident took place, yet a statement like that was like pinning a medal on a soldier's breast. It kept alive my resolution made years before.

If my battle will be in any way an inspiration to you, especially you who have fallen by the way, I shall be very happy. It is a passion with me to help others secure that wonderful feeling of physical fitness, which I have enjoyed for many years.

I am just as enthusiastic to-day and get the same inspiration out of life as I did twenty-five years ago. I have the same thirst to learn and investigate, which in my boyhood days was so unslacking. You must remember that the many years of sickness had naturally impaired my education, and I worked night and day to develop myself, mentally and physically.

The little story you read at the beginning of this chapter happened not long after I started school. Because I was weak, I was an easy prey to the other boys, who took delight in licking their smaller classmates in order to show their superiority. It must have been the blood of my father's that had lain dormant within my veins, that revolted against this treatment, and kept me coming back until I finally wiped the slate clean of all the old scores.

My ancestors have all been adventurers one way or another, and no doubt it was their blood that called me to follow the trails of adventure. On my maternal side some were pioneers of the American wilderness. Another fought through the Peninsular campaign under Sir Thomas Moore of Corunna fame, and later under Wellington, until he finally laid down his life on the field at Waterloo. The Crimea saw another who went through the slaughter of Alma, and the horrors of the night surprise at Inkerman. The Indian Mutiny, the Sudanese campaign under Kitchener, saw others of my people helping to carve history. In the more peaceful capacity of a missionary, a relative in China, with his wife and children, were included in the massacre of the Christians during the Boxer rebellion. Yet another was to be one of the successful who struggled against the elements of nature, that had conquered so many expeditions, and taken their members' lives, or made maniacs of the survivors, when they sought to lay the wires of communication across the great Australian desert. For myself, the great Northwest claimed me, with its blinding snows and freezing wastes, that resounded to the mushing of huskies and the tingle of sleigh bells, the sound of the axe and the song of the saw, and the running of the logs in spring—where man's right arm is his best weapon, and his word his bond of honor.

I have seen many strange places, and have been through many strange experiences. I have known what it is to starve and be athirst, to freeze and sleep without a roof. But maybe Jack London was right when he said, "For all that, it helps to make a man."

I don't regret any of it, but I recognize the fact that if it had not been for the many hours I devoted to exercise, I would not have been alive to-day. It built for me a sturdy body filled with vigorous stamina that overcame all physical trials, where other men fell and died.

Exercise gave me life. If I had followed the lines of least resistance like so many do, I would have died as the doctors predicted, at fifteen years of age or before, eking out each day in physical misery. Personally, I would have no kick if I died to-morrow, because I have lived more than twice the time predicted for me by our doctors and all of it in health and usefulness.

For the first time I have told of my early struggles, which will prove to you that every cloud has a silver lining, and I want to help anyone and everyone turn their particular cloud inside out, so that each can become all he wants to be physically.

No doubt some of my experiences will be of great interest to you, so I am going to recite a few, not with the desire to make believe that I am some heroic being, or Hercules come back to life, but because so many have requested it. Anyhow trials of strength are always interesting no matter how, or where, they are performed. I have not the slightest intention to tell you here of any of my athletic achievements on the platform or in the arena, but rather of feats of strength that were performed on the spur of the moment, for I believe that a strongman must be a strongman on all occasions. These stunts will have the effect of proving more conclusively to you that the right kind of exercise creates the right kind of strength, the kind that will enable you to lift the side of an automobile at a moment's notice as easily as you can lift a heavy bar bell or dumb-bell over three or four weeks of special training.

There is one particular incident I love to remember, by reason of the great bond of friendship it established between the other party and myself, friendship that has continued over the years. It happened when I was in England, when my weakness to meet strong men and look upon strange implements (made difficult to handle by reason of their awkward construction) was at its strongest pitch. Somewhere or somehow, I just cannot recall exactly, I heard some men talking about how strong they were. In the course of the conversation one of them mentioned the fact that he was willing to wager any amount that there was not one among them that could lift the "big anvil." What surprised me was the lack of interest shown. At once, I began to figure that lifting the "big anvil", as they termed it, was some test of strength very familiar to the locality. Not one of them would consider the wager. Instead, they began to razz the man who started the argument, saying that he was no sport, or he would have introduced a feat where a man had at least a sporting chance to win. Naturally I became all ears, and listening in on the talk, it seemed that

13

there was a certain blacksmith who occupied a smithy not very far from there in a small village. His great strength was proverbial. In his possession was a huge anvil that weighed, according to their talk, over thirty stone. This blacksmith stood alone in this particular feat of raising the anvil off the resting block, and no one else had ever duplicated his feat. Now as there are fourteen pounds to a stone, I figured that this anvil must weigh over four hundred and twenty pounds. It certainly had me guessing, and my anxiety to see this terrific piece of metal was tremendous. I determined that on the first opportunity I would pay the mighty smith a visit. The chance soon presented itself. One bright, beautiful spring morning, I set out to locate this remarkable son of Vulcan. I had to walk a distance of eight miles, automobiles not being so plentiful in those days, but I enjoyed every foot of the way, as the air was filled with the fragrant breath of glorious spring time. At the foot of a hill that ran into a long valley, I espied a quaint little village which I knew was my destination. However, I stopped on the outskirts of this rural hamlet to examine the beautiful structure of an old Norman church that was erected in the reign of King John of Magna Charta fame. Then to my ears came the tuneful ring of a hammer beating iron upon an anvil, which caused my pace to quicken. Arriving at the village forge, I made pretense of lingering at the door to watch the smith forge the gleaming iron upon the anvil. As I did so my eyes rested upon one of the most magnificent specimens of manhood that I have ever seen. In appearance the smith bore a striking resemblance to how our Saxon forefathers must have looked. His head seemed perfectly molded to wear the winged Viking helmet, which we visualize with our forbears, and he immediately impressed me with such an idea—tall and as straight as an arrow, with his shirt open at the throat, and sleeves rolled up he was a noble sight. He was blithely whistling a merry tune to the time of his hammer, and I thought what a carefree, happy character he was. He was powerfully constructed, and his chest seemed to swell from the throat like the crest of a wave. The neck was columnar, and he carried his head beautifully poised upon the shoulders. Arms like Longfellow's village blacksmith—bands of steel. His light brown hair swept a noble brow, from underneath which gleamed the clearest pair of blue eyes imaginable. The moment they threw their piercing gaze upon me, my soul seemed to throb with admiration. They said their cheerful day greetings to me, before the lips could repeat them. The man appealed to me tremendously, and intuition told me we were going to be friends. His cheerfulness made acquaintance easy and we talked about various things.

Almost as soon as I had entered the forge, I had espied the huge double-horned anvil set upon a large metal resting block, not far from the anvil upon which the smith was working. He noticed the way my eyes were continually being drawn in that direction, and I know he was not surprised when I walked over to look it over. I had never seen such a large anvil, and I told him so. In reply, he told me they only used it for heavy forgings and with a pleasant smile, asked me how much I thought it weighed. My reply was evasive, exclaiming that it was very hard to say but I knew it was monstrously heavy. He looked me over, and perhaps he recognized within me much of my latent strength, as he asked if I thought I could lift the anvil. I told him that I would have to be shown first how anyone else could move such an object, before I considered such an attempt. To tell the truth, I was curious to know just how he would go about it, for, heavens, it seemed a terribly unwieldy affair to handle. Laughingly he complied. Stepping forward, he caught each horn in the hollow of his arms, and with one great effort he lifted the mass off the resting block, and replaced it. With pride he said, "I am the only man that has ever lifted it clear off the block, like that." But I shocked him when I replied, "I believe I can lift it." "You can?" he questioned. "Well, I am going to try if you have no objections." I came back and as I began to take off my coat and collar he was all willingness, and cried out in admiration as he saw my well-muscled arms.

The moment I had seen him lift the anvil, I knew I could lift it, as I had proven myself capable on many occasions to sustain enormous weights in the hollow of my arms. I also knew if I could get the anvil up on my chest I could beat him in the test. Approaching the anvil, I began to apply myself to the task. Placing my feet firmly on the floor, I sought a perfect balance as I circled each horn within the fold of the elbows. I began to lift steadily, but found the anvil a little more awkward than I had anticipated. The floor of the anvil was much wider than the face, and each of the two corners nearest to my body, pressed very uncomfortably in my abdomen. However, I raised the anvil and got it resting partly upon the chest, so that it lay at a slanting angle with the floor. Leaning slightly back, I managed to support the major part of the burden upon the body. Hugging the huge piece of metal to me, I began to walk. It was a very difficult feat, as the base of the anvil was borne low enough on the hips to make any hip movement difficult. It was a terrific test, and every muscle in my body was taxed to its limit. I walked round the forge floor and then replaced the anvil on its support while I almost panted from the test. The smith looked on speechless, but coming out of his stupor with a rush, he grasped my hand and said, "You are only a boy, but you're a marvel." Well, I was only eighteen. However, he was not satisfied, for he told me "Sonny, I have never been equaled for my strength, and I am not going to say I'm beaten until it is proven in an all-round test." Right there, we pitted our strength against each other. We twisted iron and bent horseshoes. One, which may have been a little more brittle in texture than another, I broke in two. On every test I beat him, but he was a foeman worthy of any man's steel. Finally we turned wrists, in which I proved victor more easily than on any other of our previous tests. As his arm went down for the third time, he broke out into laughter. There was nothing selfish in his soul, he admired me for what I had proven myself to be that morning, and right there commenced a friendship that has endured the test of time.

Before I left that day, I gave him a photo of myself. This he nailed up on the door of a tool case that hung on the wall, and around it he nailed the two parts of the horseshoe, while over the head of the photo he nailed the stillest piece of iron I had bent. I used to visit him often while I was in England, but fifteen summers have passed since I last saw him. Yet, two or three times a year a letter creeps overseas through the mails to remind me of our pact. His children have long since grown to manhood and womanhood, but their father has taught them to remember with pride the man they can scarcely remember seeing. Last fall I received a letter, and in it the old smith said, "Your photo still hangs upon the door, with the old pieces of horseshoe and the iron you handled. Of course, the picture has faded but not your memory. When any one comes in the shop and talks about strength, the children just point to the wall and tell them that nobody could beat you."

Such faithfulness and admiration I feel keenly, because we seldom find it. The poet knew of what he was talking when he wrote the line, "True friendship is a rare jewel, and as priceless as eternity." You would be surprised if you knew some of the great strongmen I took to lift that anvil and who failed. It was a mighty test of strength.

A very amusing incident happened at one time when I lived in Canada. I happened to be in a new piece of country, where they were erecting telephone poles for wiring. The telephone operatives were a lively bunch of boys, all full of life. On this particular occasion I was lying

17

sprawled out on the grass, watching four men coming toward me, carrying a new post for erection. As they passed the foreman called out jokingly to me that if I had any excess strength that morning I could use it by helping them out, if I wished. I called back a laughing answer that the poles were too light for me, adding that if I could not raise one of them overhead with one arm, I'd eat my shirt. Like a flash they took me up, and swore I would have to eat my shirt. To their amazement I took up the bet. I began the test by centering the pole, and then I got it to the shoulder by a semi-rocking and curling process. From this stage I had no trouble at all, raising it to arms' length by using the method of the bent press. It went up beautifully. To say they were astounded, would express the situation mildly. From then on I heard the most remarkable accounts of that feat. Some said it weighed 400 pounds, and others said 500 pounds. Others with a more vivid imagination began to calculate the weight on the score that four men could easily carry 250 pounds each, so it must have weighed 1000 pounds. My estimate of the weight was about 200 pounds. I had previously weighed one and found it to weigh 185 pounds. I had performed the stunt before, and knew beforehand what I was attempting. For all that, it is a very difficult feat, as the surface is so large that the pole is apt to roll off the hand. I thoroughly enjoyed the situation, and got many a laugh from the terribly exaggerated stories that grew out of that stunt.

I have often wondered to myself if the many who hesitate to take up physical training, ever stop to realize how the various senses of fear and cowardliness give place to fortitude and confidence In the process of reconstructing the body. This was one of the first assets I recognized to spring from my training. Before, I would cringe with fear, and even go around a block rather than pass one of my tormentors, even though he would be on the opposite side of the street. So much pampering in consideration of sickness had created within me that revolting weakness of self pity. As I began to feel my feet on the ground, as it were, I refused to get out of the way for anyone. I grew confident, and with it came a degree of fairness which is so compatible with the true sportsman. I believed in being courteous and frank, and all the time grew stronger. My heart held within it a call that ever urged me, and told me I would never again know fear or be the coward I once was. I threw all those enslaving shackles off, and many have been the times when my confidence, fortitude and mental strength were demanded to a greater extent than any muscular strength. It has saved my life many times and often the lives of others.

I am so earnest in my desire to impress upon you the many values, both seen and unseen, that are obtained from a well trained physically fit body, that I want you to go with me through one of my many adventures, when confidence in oneself decided the issue of life or death.

Now please don't get into your head the idea that I always was an extraordinary brave man. That is not so. I do not esteem bravery, in most cases, as being what hero worshippers try to convey. It is only one of our natural gifts which we all possess, but like our undeveloped muscles, these senses need cultivation and stimulus. In another chapter, I will prove it again when I introduce to you, Albert Shakesby, the great, but not famous, athlete evangelist; the man who was a match for Hackenschmidt, the man who outlifted—now I am digressing in my enthusiasm, so let me get back and take you through the adventure that chills me to the bone whenever I think of it.

Just previous to this little adventure I had made the acquaintance of a husky seaman, who had the same passions as myself to see things. He had heard that eighteen miles from where we had docked, lay the remains of a once prosperous fishing town. It appeared that during the days of the buccaneers this town was an ideal resort for them, on

19

account of its natural harbor, point of prominence, and general inaccessibility. According to history its people had always been engaged in freebooting. I remember on our visit seeing the remains of an old lighthouse, that was a couple of miles inland from where it should have been, and many harrowing stories are told about ships that were lured to destruction by the wreckers. Morgan and the notorious Captain Kidd had used this place of refuge at one time or another; but the place of interest was the natural cavern, which was jealously kept a secret for generations and named after Robin Lythe, a very early freebooter. We set off on foot together, early in the day, arriving at our destination some time about high noon. We were rather dismayed when we saw the great difficulties that faced us, and which had to be overcome if we wanted to see the object of our desire. The harbor was a natural cleft cut into the cliffs like a bight. It was strewn with rocks, and the cave entrance was away out on the face of the cliff that fronted the sea. Nobody would let us have a boat, but after coming so far, we were determined that we were not going back without making some attempt to see this cave. We decided to climb our way out on the side of the cliff, after being informed that the tide was never low enough to allow walking to the site of this notorious place. Taking off our shoes and socks, we tied the laces, and slung them over our shoulders. It was some climb, believe me. One misstep would have plunged us to our death upon the jagged rocks beneath, around which continually swirled the hungry eddies. Climbing thus for almost an hour, we came to the entrance. By walking on the various ledges that gave us foothold, we entered. It was a beautiful sight. The walls seemed to be all colors, constantly changing, and the water was naturally calm but had a swift current. In many places we were obliged to almost double up, and the farther we went in the darker it became. Many were the bumps we sustained against the low roof. We finally traversed the cavern, which I would describe as more of a passage, and with great relief we stepped out upon the sands. Lying down to rest from our laborious, dangerous climb, our eyes began to rove around our surroundings. We had come to a hollow of the cliff that reminded me of an amphitheatre. Circular, the cliffs rose high and straight. On observation it was easy to see what an impregnable retreat this had been. We looked around, but were unable to find a point in the cliff that was scalable. The cliffs rose to a height of over 200 feet. We quickly tired of our searching, which disclosed nothing more interesting than the remains of a dead monkey, an old high boot, some old cooking utensils and broken boxes. These were in other caves that were naturally cut into the cliff and no doubt used by the pirates as eating and sleeping quarters. Our ambitions satisfied, and well pleased with our adventure we started to find our way out. To our consternation, when we approached the passage we found the tide had risen. In our eagerness we had never thought of this condition. It was impossible to negotiate, as it was almost closed with the rising water. Previously we had found the walls unscalable, and we realized that we were trapped. What other method of egress the former occupants had, had been demolished, or naturally closed up by the shifting sands. We had to do some quick thinking before the floor of the amphitheatre was covered. I figured that a place so alive with cavities might possibly have some that went right through the cliff and penetrated into the harbor. I explained to my companion that the pirates would never have overlooked such an asset, the only trouble was whether the passage was entirely negotiable or not. For such a place, we looked. In our search we came to a small passage at the foot of the cliff that would just permit the body of a man, lying flat, to enter. I explained that here was our only chance, but my friend could not see it. He argued that it took me all my time to squeeze in when investigating and once we were in we might never get out. I argued that was the chance we had to take, and I was going to make the attempt no matter what he did. I began the passage. Lying flat upon my body I wriggled in, with arms stretched out in front of my head. It was terribly dark, and some parts were so narrow that my body was cut in many places. The air was suffocating, and I was quickly bathed in perspiration. I began to feel that I was choking from the stifling air and tried to back out, but as I did, my pull-over sweater was caught by the jagged rock roof of the passage. I realized I was trapped. Like a flash, the fear of dying like a drowned rat, or of suffocation shot through my mind, and a cold sweat gathered across my brow. It created panicky thoughts, but immediately I suppressed them and began to tell myself that if I had a chance to win, it could only be won by keeping cool. So my only chance lay in going ahead. I began to congratulate myself on not having neglected deep breathing and chest development. I certainly felt the value of good lungs in that congested space.

Inch by inch, I wormed onward. Some places were so narrow I had a terrible time squeezing by. Then other parts lacked depth, and I was obliged to paw the sand away. It was as black as pitch and terribly noisome. The sound of my labored breathing seemed to beat in the drums of my ears. I struggled onward with set lips. Then like a God-send, I felt the current of cool air. It raised my hopes. Then I saw a tiny light. How I struggled toward it, I can never describe. Every inch of the way was a battle until I came to the outlet and felt the salt spray beat against my face. I lay panting for breath, happily allowing the fresh air and salt water to saturate my being. Then I thought of my friend, I saw no time was to be lost as the incoming tide would soon close this only hope. Again I had to negotiate that awful trip, but I did it with a song in my heart. I found my friend terribly distressed; but even when I showed him the only way out, he flatly refused to make the passage. My clothes were torn and I was bleeding, and my eyes were bloodshot from the sifting sand. Finally I told him if he would not go with me, I would leave him, as I had no notion of dying unnecessarily. When he saw I was determined to leave him, he began to follow. Well, if my other two passages were trials, this last trip was worse. He almost went crazy. It is all right for some people to laugh when they hear of such a trial, and say what they would do, and all that, but they were never in such a place. Talk is cheap. I have run the gauntlet of steel and bullets more than once, and one time, with a companion, fought for four hours in a boat to break loose from the grip of a dangerous whirlpool. But then, we could see what we were doing, and we had more excitement to spur us on. Here it was like entering blindly a tomb in the bowels of the earth.

I had to keep talking to encourage my friend, and all the time he hung onto one of my feet. Once or twice it slipped from his grasp, and he almost went frantic, screaming for me not to leave him. The sound of his voice in that space was head-splitting, but finally we got out. I don't know how long it took us, but it seemed to be an eternity. The next thing for which we were to be thankful was that we had been seen making our climb out around the cliff side. The fishermen knew the conditions and had become alarmed for our safety and were out looking for us. They were amazed to see us crawl out of the hole in the side of the cliff, bleeding and exhausted, and glad we were to be dragged into the boat and be taken ashore.

My companion was physically a better man than the average. He had proven himself so on various occasions, but he fell down here. Of course, any one might have done the same, but what I am getting at is the fact that he recognized that it meant a lot to know your own capabilities. He recognized that training of mind and of the body was a natural co-ordination, and increased the efficiency of a man.

Some of you who read this may say that you will never have to face such a circumstance. Well, I sincerely hope you will not, yet you never know what you may have to face. It was not long ago that thousands of men were drawn from peaceful walks of life, to be thrown into the maelstrom and horrors of war. It was the man who knew himself who made out the best! and the psychologists, and others who had charge of our national destiny, knew that physical training was the one thing that best equipped the soldier to meet all emergencies.

If a man is capable of meeting the extreme test with fortitude, he certainly will be more efficient to meet minor tests. Most weaklings are cowards, because they lack the material with which to back up their will.

Just sit down a few moments and question yourself honestly. Search your heart thoroughly, and I am sure you will agree with me that there is much to be improved in yourself. Even if you are athletic, you can never keep up the standard of fitness unless you stick to a few minutes of practice. It amply repays you for the time spent.

I never regret the many hours devoted to this practice. It meant a new lease of life to me, and as I draw this chapter to a close let me say that such splendid specimens of humanity as Sandow, Maxick, and Pullum all traversed the same road to secure what they got. They were not miracles, although it may appear so. Just remember them, and let their lives inspire you, as I was inspired. Everybody has the same chance, and the man who is normally healthy, really, has no obstacles to face.

Perseverance, patience and determination will be repaid in untold wealth, health, strength, self-reliance and fortitude.

CHAPTER II
THE TRUTH ABOUT EXERCISE

It takes all kinds of people to make a world, but some we often feel should be given an island, to make a world of their own. There are people who apparently are born with the pessimistic germ in their systems. They just cannot help taking a contrary view of the situation. You find them everywhere, and antagonistic to the popular beliefs of life, law and religion. I agree that the major part of their criticism is destructive rather than constructive, but why worry about them if you know you are right. You may say, "Look at the harm they do." But I do not believe that. Like attracts like is my belief. Some people prefer to believe that black is white, so let them believe it. We have the same spirit to contend with in teaching the valuable precepts of physical training. I happened to know a man who had an argumentative belief that exercise was harmful; he accosted a heart specialist on the question, with whom I am familiar. The specialist informed him that the causes of cardiac conditions were reduced to four, none of which were caused by exercise. The only time sports or exercise are liable to injure the heart are when the heart is out of condition. Then anything would injure it. More often bad eating, but rarely right exercise, which is constructive. The other man replied that just the same he believed exercise hurts the heart. Now a wall would have to fall on such a man before he would believe it had fallen. And, as an angel could not convert such a person, why worry about it?

If you believe in statistics only, then we find the Harvard University reports are convincing proof that exercise and athletics are greatly beneficial in improving the body and preserving longevity. The report reads that if there is any effect upon the health, the effect is beneficial. How can it be otherwise. A machine will rust from non-use more quickly than it will wear out, and the same explanation stands good for the body. The muscles deteriorate with non-use. If they stopped with their own deterioration it would be bad enough, but unfortunately the internal organs become bereft of their protection, which places them in the same class as the soldier without his steel helmet. The truth of exercise lies in the value it accumulates, and like a steadily growing bank account, it develops an earning power. No logical minded person disapproves of putting a little bit away for a rainy day. If a horticulturist has an attractive bloom he does not forget to water it, and till the soil that surrounds the plant to fertilize the roots. The key thought is cultivation. If you have any good talent you cultivate it to preserve and make it more effective. If it is not as good as it should be, you study how to make it so by careful cultivation. Exercise is just another term for cultivation. By cultivating the body you prolong its usefulness. Some say that once exercise is commenced, it has to be kept up. Well, now, you never see the thrifty individual draw upon his financial resources, or the horticulturist forget his bloom, or the owner of an apiary forget his bees. Then what reason should there be for a person to neglect what he has. The battle is always to the strong, and the "survival of the fittest" is based upon how long the individual can retain his superiority over the rest. The same law is in existence, but in a more cultured sense, and as it claims a natural origin, it must have a natural existence. The mere theory of a man cannot change the fundamentals of the natural law, which demand preservation or consignment to the junk pile.

There is a religion attached to body culture which is every bit the equal of soul culture. Longfellow wrote that "the voice was the organ of the soul." Equally so is the body the expression of your life and living. You must remember that there is all the difference in the world between being born right and living right. Nature may have been very bountiful at birth, but if neglect to preserve what was inherited comes with the succeeding years, then that individual is doomed to fall by the wayside. Some of our finest examples of physical cultivation were unfortunate in not being born right, but they lived right. These men recognized the fact that exercise held a truth, so they followed it. Clean living, right living, or truthful living, whatever you want to call it, will not stand for any dictation from man. You are the one who must obey. One of the great Christian prophets admonished man to "Keep sacred the body, even as the soul," and another instructs us "The body is the holy temple of the soul." It is not my intention to discuss religion, beyond that of the body. It is merely my desire to prove to any who may be skeptical that the merits of body culture have always been considered on a par with soul culture. The Platonic age of Greece was only created by the study and universal acceptance of body culture, and that state only disappeared when they began to neglect those principles.

The biggest obstacle to the mind of the average layman is to determine the best method of exercise. Of course we hear a lot of different beliefs and they all hold a certain amount of truth. The greatest benefit of exercise, as I see it, is not in merely doing just this and that to keep normally fit for the day, as much as it is in the creative value of storing up energies within ourselves to meet the approaching years with all the vitality of youth, so far as this is possible. This being the object, what we should look for is the method that is naturally going to give us the best results with the least expenditure of time. I cannot see the value of training two or three hours every night, or making every bodily movement a physical exercise, when intensive training for about thirty minutes every other night will do better. It is proven that it does better. A method that involves numerous repetitions is not apt to be intensive, and the "every movement physical" idea involves a nervous depletion if

27

carried too far. In either case, no natural gains are registered in the store room of physical energy. We know that muscles must have strength, and strength is another name for ability to overcome resistance. The muscles must have resistance to stimulate their motive powers. There is an old saying that "Strength begets Strength." Such being the case, it is only logical that strength methods should be used. You cannot use strength without resistance, and this resistance must be intensive, simply because the muscles are built to more than take care of the body, so it is only logical to substitute weights to give the additional resistance. The progressive weight policy is to coax the muscles, and give the weight increase with the proportionate increase of strength, and not to exert all the power in one or two struggling efforts. It is lack of facts that gives some people that illogical idea. The strange part to me is the lack of balance we see in some people. They may be very sincere, but when you see them struggling to the point of fatigue, trying to chin themselves a number of times and then hear them say that progressive bar bell methods are too strenuous, it cannot help but raise a smile. For at no time will a bar bell user misapply his power in one whole session like the chinning fiend, who never thinks of building his body up proportionately in order to make him more efficient for that test. Others argue that weight lifters strain themselves when lifting. If one does, he is better fitted to do so than any other athlete, because he develops all his powers. He always has a respite between each lift and the lifts are few and quickly done. None are the protracted exertions displayed by the runner and sculler. You never saw a weight-lifter collapse during a contest, or at the close of one, as is frequently the case with runners and scullers, and it is a proven fact that weight-lifters recuperate faster than any other athletes. This subject is not by the way, it merely goes to prove that if weight-lifting as a sport does not entail greater exertions than other sports, it proves how safe bar bell training is for body building purposes. It is vastly superior to the routine of a chinning or dipping fiend. The bar bell athlete has the study of muscular economy brought down to a science, and the value of distribution is evident to a greater degree because one group of muscles are not developed at the expense of another, as in other sports. Intensive exercise develops all the muscles. I have heard field coaches disapprove of the body builder who shows an outstanding development of all his muscles, but just get him talking about some of his track stars, and he will point with pride to the legs of his sprinters, the shoulders of the hammer throwers, and the arms of the shot putter. I do not believe in specializing on one group of muscles to make a man efficient at one sport only. Such a body is like a one track mind. Muscular team work is what delights one, and it is because the bar bell exerciser has the finest team muscles of all athletes that he is the best all round man. He certainly is the strongest and the most supple, which makes him a capable weight-lifter, wrestler, hand balancer and tumbler. He has every bit as much stamina and endurance as the marathon runner, and is not as liable to fatigue. As a jumper, he can meet them all despite the heavier bodyweight handicap. There are Willoughby, Kingsbury, Betty, Bevan, Levan, Berry, Coulter, Gauss, Hoffman, Steinborn, Marineau, Fournier, Gorner, Cadine, Miller, Londos and a host of other crack bar bell men I can mention, who are superb swimmers, jumpers, shot putters, hammer throwers, scullers, boxers, wrestlers and many of them are ten second men in the hundred yard dash. Show me a boxer or a man who concentrates on track events or who relied upon methods of training, other than the intensive system as supplied by bar bells, as accomplished as the bar bell athlete.

Some wise critic said that it took two blows of a boxer to put out a wrestler, and one for a weight-lifter. That makes me laugh. What would the boxer say if we were to put it this way. The lifter will lift fifty percent more than a strong wrestler, and three times more with one hand than a boxer will do with two hands. Right away, he would say that was the lifter's game. Well, it is a poor man who can't beat another at his own game, but make it a rough and tumble fight, a free for all, and the best boxer is hopelessly beaten. I have seen on more than one occasion, a world's champion thrashed by third rate rough and tumble men. The sport of lifting weights is so closely allied to bar bell exercise because we are enabled by it to test the value of the progress made, in much the same manner as a sprinter finds the improvement in his start, stride and finish, cuts down his time over the hundred yards.

I have often seen reference made to the great strength of porters and baggage men in handling big trunks, etc., but that is mostly a question of counterpoise rather than strength, although there is undoubtedly a certain amount of strength involved. I know that a husky weight lifter or a bar bell exercise fan, with a little practice, will easily exceed the professional porter. There is less comparison between a lumberjack and a porter than we have been taught. There is less chance of employing counterpoise in handling logs than there is in handling trunks.

If it was dangerous to exercise at all, and particularly on the intensive system, it would be dangerous to make any kind of a lift. Go back into history and you will read where barbaric races terrified the Romans by the huge rocks they hurled upon them. It was a pastime of the ancient Gauls to compete in raising the largest stone overhead with both hands and throw it the greatest distance. Actually the progressive principle dates further back than the story of Milo of Croton. A friend of mine who is a great student of Egyptology and has been a member of various research and excavation parties, in Egypt, told me that in one tomb they came across a miniature plate loading bar bell made in wood. On the other hand, we find the Chinese, whose dynasties date further into antiquity than those of Assyria or Chaldee, retain a peculiar ancient custom that probably dates from Confucius. Piled up in a part of the town or village are a series of stone bar bells, each one weighing more than the other until a certain weight is reached. It is the Chinese custom for the young man to graduate in this lifting school before he can claim to have reached manhood.

The human race is naturally progressive, and when nature outlines the method of progress it must be right, and as we have full evidence of the natural method of progression in developing the physical state, the progressive method of intensive training, as practiced today on a more scientific basis, must be right. Perhaps it is this natural method of physical progression that has improved our physical state that has brought forward the statement from scientists that the modern man is healthier than the ancients. Further investigation proves to us the great possibilities to which a human being can develop his strength by following the same natural law, providing you are willing to recognize the abilities of some races who apply themselves to manual work more than we do.

Let us consider the main method of transportation in and around Constantinople, and over the Balkans as carried out by the Armenians. A certain body of these men form what we would call a Guild, and among this Balkan race it is a very ancient order. It is composed of none others but carriers, who do all the transporting of supplies. The amount of weight some of these men carry day in and day out on their back is almost incredible, I have seen them walk along the streets of Constantinople of times with a crier going in advance of them for the privilege of the road to which they are entitled. Their legs almost seem to bow under the load upon their back, which is anywhere from six hundred pounds to one thousand pounds. I saw the report of an American resident of the suburb of Constantinople, who reported an amazing incident in his diary. He had ordered five tons of coal to be delivered to his suburban home, and to his surprise the delivery was made by five men who each made two trips, which would run them about one thousand pounds a trip for each load. On the Isle of Cyprus is an order of monks, who among other things have dedicated their lives to perform everything by manual labor. They hitch themselves to the plow to cultivate the soil and have been known to carry loads varying from five hundred and sixty pounds to nine hundred and fifty pounds upon their backs at one time. They are endowed with remarkable physiques and are long lived. Why some should be so insistent in promoting the belief that people who exercise die young, is ridiculous to me, when statistics show otherwise. They pick out a few athletes who have died rather prematurely, but they never advance the statistics that show the terrible percentage of men who die in their twenties and thirties from preventable diseases. What are a few solitary exceptions against a multitude of facts? We have no way of knowing how long those few athletes who die young would have lived if they had never taken up the study of body culture. Most of them that I know of died of neglect. It is a fact that is recognized by insurance companies that athletes do not take sufficient care of themselves. They think because they are so strong they can overcome everything and never give in until it is too late. Such was the case of Arthur Saxon. After the war was over, from which he had already suffered, he joined a carnival giving numerous shows daily. It was here he contracted pneumonia by exposure and negligence during inclement weather, and in this state he tried to go on day by day with his act, refusing to throw a robe over his shoulders between the other acts despite his weakness and profuse perspiration. A strong man who was with him at that time told me that Saxon actually died on his feet.

Breitbart died of septic poisoning. He tore his leg on a nail and went on daily with his act, scorning treatment. After he contracted this dreadful sickness, he actually lived three weeks, which is an unheard of circumstance, as septic poisoning is supposed to kill in about twenty-four hours. When his life could have been saved by amputating his leg, he refused.

Sandow had no kick coming. The best medical specialists in Europe only gave him eighteen years to live, and he survived until he was sixty. When he died, it was as the result of an automobile accident.

The government of the United States spends huge sums of money annually to promote the teachings of physical training throughout the schools, army and the navy. Universities and colleges consider the subject of physical education a very important part of a student's learning, and everything is done to encourage a student to devote time to cultivate his body as well as his mind. Since this system has been fostered the statistics from the universities and colleges have been able to show a higher rating for every student both mentally and physically. These facts must prove to the most skeptical that if these great institutions find physical training such a vital part of a person's education, to such an extent that they spend millions of dollars annually, there must be some greater value attached to exercise than is generally conceded. If exercise was merely a whim with no apparent value, it is a certainty that the government and these other institutions would not consider it. If it was dangerous to the individual they would quickly crush the movement altogether. Commander Byrd, who led the MacMillan Arctic expedition and who recently flew over the North Pole, realized the necessity of keeping his crew and himself physically fit. On each of these Arctic expeditions, Commander Byrd wrote to me asking me to supply them with the necessary equipment and instructions. Intensive training on the progressive bar bell plan was practiced by these hardy adventurers as a necessary part of their plans to keep them fit in order to help clinch success in their hazardous undertaking.

Exercise can be better understood as man building. The benefits accumulated are not just physical, they are manifold. The mental and organic system are developed along with the nervous and physical system, and the senses are all intensified. I mean the co-ordinating senses that control confidence and reliance, which all must be considered as part of the quota that goes to make a man one hundred percent physically efficient. There is no "open Sesame" to body culture. Everybody has to work for what they get and by their efforts will their results be measured. The young man who thinks he can burn the candle at both ends is going to regret it. Youth has an abundance of buoyant vitality, but this should be conserved and not expended. Because fools rush in where angels fear to tread, is no reason why another should think it safe to emulate them! because of youth being on their side. The days when "wild oats" were supposed to have been a necessary part of a young man's education has long since passed away. We live in the age of doing things, where the great lesson is conservation and the ability to meet emergencies and still carry on. Reserve is needed and this must be the ammunition supply of the body like the bandolier for the rifle. The truth of all these things lies in the proper understanding of exercise. In the following chapters I am giving you the truthful fruits of my knowledge and investigation of exercise, so that you can put them to good account and be another successful exponent of man building.

CHAPTER III
DEFINING THE MYSTERY OF STRENGTH

There seems to be some mystery that surrounds the meaning of strength, insomuch as the average individual finds it very difficult to explain. The general way of figuring strength runs something like this: A baseball fan knows Babe Ruth must be strong to be able to swat a ball for so many home runs, and that Johnson, Washington's star pitcher, must have a strong arm to send the pill hurtling over the plate with such terrific force. Charlie Hoff and Charlie Paddock are strong by reason of the great leg driving force possessed by each. However, these cases are purely demonstrations of strength, and not definitions. When you ask for the explanation of the strength of a man who is capable of raising a big load on his back, or tossing a dumb-bell to arms' length overhead, the answer is partly explained, in the absence of a broader knowledge, by the fact that the person must have been naturally barn strong.

These few answers prove how very little is known about the most desirable quality of a man's body, and bring us face to face with the question of whether all strong people are always naturally strong, or if it is possible to be made strong—the difference between natural strength and made strength, if there is any, and the relation of health to strength.

I have a friend who has a very analytical mind, and he just loves to produce a difficult problem to be solved. He is not one of the kind who do it to show how much they know, or think they know, as much as he is naturally curious to know the answer for his own benefit. If it is beyond him, it bothers him considerably. The question of strength was one of his problems, and I well recall the time when he asked me if it was true that we could make strength. Now if any other person but he had asked me, I would have answered yes; but all his questions place me on my guard, and after a pause I replied that I had my doubts. This, no doubt, will cause my readers to scratch their heads in consternation, as I am well aware that some theorists have brought forward the statement that strength can be made, and that there are two kinds of strength, natural strength and made strength; but the distinction never grew to be believed in because no proper separation of the two kinds of strength is possible. We have a habit of saying that a certain person was made strong by practicing exercise or some particular sport, but that does not mean to say his strength was made. Strength is the outcome of certain causes, and like gravity, or the bloom of a flower, it cannot be disassociated from its natural condition. If it was possible to control strength and disassociate it from muscular growth, as it is possible to separate muscular growth of a certain nature from strength, we might consider the fact that possibly strength could be made. It is the existence of the type of muscle that lacks strength which causes the difference between size and strength to be too often misunderstood.

You have often seen young men who possessed a fine muscular appearance, that apparently had every indication of strength. Yet, on a test, you have been amazed to see that these particular parties were seldom any stronger than the average man. Then there is the other type of man who, while possessing no larger proportions than the first, was capable of moving objects that were immovable to both the first named type and the average person.

It is a mystery that has led theorists to state that muscle was all artificial, and that there was some "nigger in the wood pile" where strength was concerned.

Now there is a great deal of difference in the construction of muscle tissue, and the student of body culture should be made familiar with the structure of muscle in order to better understand its true existence, and the interpretation of strength. Therefore, before we go any further, we will supply ourselves with the knowledge which tells us what it is all about. Then we will realize why strength is an inseparable part of one type of muscle, and why it can never be associated with the other type.

First, bear in mind that there are about five hundred and twenty muscles in our physical makeup that have to do with the transporting of our body. Each of these muscles are made up of thousands of little fibers that lie side by side, much like the fibers in a rope. These fibers are capable of contracting on the same order as a stretched rubber cable contracts when the tension is released. Each of these fibers has a cell or a brain, which answers the call of the true brain through the transmission of nerves, that causes them to contract or relax just as the order demands. The condition of the muscle lies in the construction of these fibers. Some methods of exercise bring about a coarse tissue, while other methods bring about a steel-like construction where the fibers become more numerous and compact.

Now, whenever anyone part of the body is under a greater stress of physical stimulation than the rest, it is a natural condition that the blood is drawn away from other parts of the body where the blood is temporarily less required, and drawn in greater quantities to the area under active stimulation. The blood contains nourishment that re-fuels the muscles in their state of activity, besides carrying away all the broken down tissue that is thrown off by the exertion, as well as cleaning out the muscle cells of any carbon dioxide that may have secreted within these cells. It also acts as a fertilizer in the process of muscular reconstruction, by reason of the fact that the blood continues to circulate around the center of activity, after the actual action has ceased.

Now get the following explanation perfectly correct in your mind. It is not in all motions of muscular activity that muscle tissue is broken down. The movements have to be intense, and the muscles must be supplied with the resistance that is necessary in order to break down the old structure.

Movements, or exercises, that do not give the muscles the required resistance, but are the kind that involve a great number of repetitions, never break down any amount of tissue, to speak of. These movements involve a forcing process, that causes the blood to swell up the muscles, and simply pumps them up. Thus a coarse tissue is created, that quickly loses its proportions unless the muscle culturists practice continually. In the other case, the muscles are supplied with a resistance, through weights, that causes full contraction and extension of the muscles, as well as a great flexion of the joints, which altogether rapidly breaks down the old structure and commences its process of reconstruction. Not many movements are involved because the motions are almost wholly physical. By this I mean the muscles do not call for a fraction of the nervous energies which is the case in the other instance.

Followers of bar bell exercise find that, before they notice any signs of increase in their proportions, they have become quite a bit stronger. The reason for this is that the musculature possessed in the first place has passed through a stage of conversion, in which this tissue has become converted into one hundred per cent material. The outcome of the other condition is what I term inflated tissue of the balloon type. They register no change in strength simply because the methods they use are not productive of strength. The fact that strength has become manifest in the latter state is positive proof that the condition created is the most natural and must, therefore, contain the properties that are productive of great strength, in both appearance and demonstration.

We have no control over strength alone. It is the natural outcome of substantial muscular growth. It can only be stimulated, and this stimulus must come from growth by development supplied from intensive exercise.

In speaking of strength, I really believe that we are apt to consider its meaning in super terms. Anyhow, it is as such I want my readers to consider it. It is in its super state that we are able to appreciate it better, and if it did not have this exalted state, we would feel all our labors were in vain, with no recompense for them. Again, if that state could not be reached, it would not provide the lesson in which we are interested.

One strange peculiarity in muscle growth is the manner in which it multiplies in its process of reconstruction, which goes to prove how nature is prepared to take care of her children and is a factor to prove my story. To continue, let me say that it is pretty hard for the average person to understand why these tissues are broken down, and when they rebuild, why they grow in excess of what they formerly were. Muscular tissues of the body fulfill their duties, wear out, and are cast off like the dead leaves of a plant, and just as the plant grows stronger, as a greater abundance of foliage appears, equally so does muscle reconstruction act. Growth is life, and life is growth; when growth ceases the body begins to age and finally dies. As tissue is broken down, it multiplies and we become stronger with growth. In other words, nature creates size, and strength is the natural sequence. Size and strength are accumulated to meet possible future necessities in excess of any work previously performed.

Let us prove this condition in another way, and be satisfied that I am right. You, no doubt, can call to mind some fellow acquaintance who went into the lumber camp, or on some railroad construction job, and how on his return his changed appearance struck you as remarkable!—how he had filled out, and how much stronger he was than before. Well, isn't that an illustration of how natural growth takes place to fulfill the requirements of a more laborious occupation?

The year after the close of the war I took a notion to take another trip overseas. I went into the Canadian Pacific Steamship offices in Montreal to purchase my ticket. I was taken care of by a clerk who had his sleeves rolled up to the shoulders. He displayed a fine pair of arms, and right away I recognized those little traits that inform a trained eye that this magnificent pair of arms was not always in his possession. He was too consciously proud of them. By his "return button" I saw he had served overseas, and to satisfy my personal curiosity, I began to question him. I had to smile at his boyish enthusiasm as he replied, "I just had to have 'em. I was with one of the batteries, and had the job of trundling heavy shells in a wheelbarrow. By gosh, at first I thought my back would break. My knees wobbled, and I felt as though each of my arms was being pulled from its socket. But, it had to be done, and I got better at it and began to like it. Pushing that wheelbarrow full of shells just made me over." "And believe me," he added with pride, "my legs and back are every bit as well formed as my arms." No doubt you will recognize this incident as a common occurrence, but it serves to prove that strength is always the result of a certain condition, and not made in the sense that we are using this word.

If it was possible for you to cut into the living muscular structure of inflated tissue and natural tissue, you would find the difference in construction much similar in appearance to the difference that is seen in the grain of cedar wood, as against the grain of oak. One is coarse grained, and the other is tight. Try to break off an oak sapling and you will find it very difficult, but a cedar sapling, twice the size, will snap off much more easily. The condition of structure and resistance is the same here as the quality of musculature under discussion.

Inflated tissue is artificial, which is borne out by the fact that this tissue lacks lasting quality and has never been productive of strength. Strength is never artificial. It is too natural, therefore its existence must arise from the creation of a natural source.

Now you are apt to get all balled up if you have not read all this material studiously, and I want it to be perfectly clear in your mind. So to condense the whole discussion to a few words, as to what it all means, we find that strength as a distinct and separate product cannot be made; it is the result of developing musculature in its natural form. We know inflated tissue does not contain this essential, but we do know that there is a form of tissue that can be developed, that does create strength. In other words, the muscular structure can be made.

As I have previously stated, intensive resistance of the muscles is the method of muscular contraction, by reason of its natural function, that can bring about the change. Therefore, it is just a case of following the right method of exercise that can produce this type of muscle.

In order to receive confirmation in any belief, let us see how the first examples of strength got their supply. I think I can safely say that I have come in contact with as many strong men as any other man, by reason of my travels and studies that have extended over twenty years, as a practical athlete. I have known thousands, and without one single exception every man instinctively practiced bar bell exercises on the progressive principle. Thousands of times I have asked if they thought that that kind of training was responsible for their fine development and great strength. Not one of them ever repudiated the weights. They were tremendously emphatic in their statements that no other form of exercise could possibly give the degree of strength that they owned. Well, you will agree with me that they ought to know. They had tried everything, and spoke from experience. No man is fool enough to practice what he knows is wrong after he has found the answer to his problem. With all this mass of testimonials behind my assertion I must be right. More so, since it completely balances with my deductions and the way we all know that nature works.

I do not ask any man to accept any of my beliefs, if I cannot prove them. Likewise any one is foolish to believe any statement at all that cannot provide the satisfactory proof, and the teacher himself is a fitting example of what he teaches.

In all my life I have never seen a strong man who was not healthy, but I have met many healthy men who were not strong. The stronger a man, the more vigorous his health, and his body retains its youth and preservation in life longer by far than the man who is healthy and yet not strong. A great number of people would have us believe that strong people become terribly muscle bound. Now nature never does anything wrong, and strength never created such a condition as muscle binding. The term is just another that is wrongly used. There are a number of muscle fans who have a mania to possess a pair of large biceps, or huge pectoral muscles. All their efforts are thrown into the exercises that will develop either of these conditions, and the trouble is that their development becomes unbalanced and exists at the expense of the rest of their bodies. Thus do other muscles become robbed of their rights and remain in a weaker condition. Not until the muscle fan has acquired this state does he realize how wrong it is, but he has no one else to thank for it except himself. No teacher of body culture ever advised it. Fortunately it is a condition that can easily be overcome by a little specialization that will recover the balance between the various muscles.

Allow me to put before you one of my latest proofs of this. Not long ago a young man, who is well known in muscle building circles, and who possesses apparently a very imposing physique, came to me and said, "How is it,

Mr. Jowett, that I am no good at lifting weights? I have the development, but lots of lighter men can easily beat me, and I can't understand it." Frankly he admitted that the circumstances had become very acute and embarrassing, due to the fact that he was not able to maintain his prestige. He was troubled because too many were telling him he would never be strong and that his muscular structure was inflated. I had seen him stripped various times and I informed him that his condition was merely one of unbalanced proportions, which I could quickly remedy; more so in his case than in most others because he had the foundation. I pointed out his weak points and showed him the best exercises to overcome his defects, and in one week he had put over one inch on his thighs (his least developed part), and lifted a weight overhead he never thought was possible. Only weighing one hundred and forty-five pounds, he performed the lift known as the Two Hands Clean and Jerk, using two hundred and twenty-five pounds. He was also capable of raising the front of an automobile, to his great delight. Some improvement, you will agree, when you remember he was miles away from these two feats a week before.

Some men are naturally born much stronger than others, for physical reasons or inheritance, but no man ever possessed the amount of natural strength that placed him in the class of such giants of strength as Cyr, Saxon or Apollon. These men were, all three, naturally strong, but it was exercise with weights on the progressive principle that increased their natural powers, stimulating their strength to a degree that enabled them to lift such terrific poundages. It is ridiculous to believe that if Saxon had never trained he would still have been able to lift overhead four hundred and forty-eight pounds. On the other hand, we have men like Sandow, Tofolas, Maxick and Pullum, four men who were deprived of the natural blessing at birth which clothed Cyr, Saxon and Apollon, but by intensive training they created from themselves supermen. My own case is another example that goes to prove, along with the other four named celebrities, that the creation of substantial muscular tissue is the substance from which great strength is derived.

Spencer, in his "Growth and Development," proves the natural condition of what I have stated, and he had no knowledge of muscle building; but he knew nature. He knew strength came from vigorous growth. You can see it in animal and plant life, just the same as in human life.

All the men to whom I have referred were capable of proving their strength in any way you wished to test them. Why people fool themselves into believing that the strength of such men only works in one direction, is positively ridiculous. As I have proven, there is only one kind of strength, and that is natural strength. Whether it is born in a man or stimulated by training under intensive exercise, it is just the same and cannot be changed; whether it is capable of applying its qualities in tossing bar bells, moving pianos, or lifting the end of an automobile out of a rut.

A man who resorts to tricks and the use of mechanical devices as an aid to perform his feats, is never strong, no matter what he says he is or how he impresses the mind. The few men whom I have named would scorn the mention of such false methods. It is the work of such tricksters that has given rise to the belief, so prevalent in many quarters, that trickery is connected with great feats of strength. There is no connection at all between the two. A strong man is always strong, no matter on what he is tested. His musculature is substantial and possesses strength which he has created within himself. Earlier in this chapter, I state that this type of structure can be made. However, there is another very important part connected with this growth which I have purposely reserved until the last, simply because I did not want to crowd you. By now you will have thoroughly absorbed all I have written, and be properly prepared for what I have to say. This explanation will clear up the question which no doubt still lingers in your mind, that causes you to wonder if the one man has secured the right material, surely the other must be able to obtain some increase of power worthwhile. Your mind questions that there must be some strength in all that muscular size. However, there never can be unless they turn to intensive training. Although the substantial material is formed, it is not exactly in that structure where the power lies. It has a co-ordinating factor that really makes powerful efforts possible, and this factor is the ligaments. The muscles are the engines of the body and the ligaments the pulleys. It is these ropes of connection that make it possible to apply the muscles in their greatest contraction. The more muscular fibers in a muscle, the more steel-like their quality, and they are capable of greater contraction. But if these ropes of connection are not strong enough to withstand the resistance required, then their weakness is evident. Because these two cannot be separated is the sole reason why strength is never disassociated from substantial structure. Ligaments always exhibit their quality by their thickness. As the right kind of muscle is formed, they become thicker. Just look at the joints of a real strong man, and note the depth of tissue that exists. Feel for the ligaments and you will notice how thick and cordy they are, but you never note their appearance on one who is not strong, or on the athlete who has not practiced bar bell exercise. When I started heavy exercise my wrist measured seven inches, but today it measures eight and a half inches. The ligaments are very thick and prominent, and have an appearance that immediately tells the eye they must be part of a sturdy combination.

Strength is better understood as resistance:—The power to resist the resistance of some other object. The muscles are continually pulling, never pushing. One group relaxes and another contracts.

There is no mystery to strength, it is just simply understanding its definition. It has a natural source, and the only thing left is for the muscle builder to cultivate that source by the right method of training—the kind that has produced the most powerful men in the world in all classes, irrespective of whether they were born strong or not. Material resistance methods, which can only be supplied by progressive bar bell training, are the only methods which can secure the desired outcome—great natural strength.

CHAPTER IV
CURATIVE EXERCISES

Broken in health, in spirit, and financially, without a single hope for the future. Nothing but pain, sleepless nights, and a nauseating terror of food. The absolute necessity of a mother to turn bread winner in order that food and clothing could be provided for two little tots who were beginning to feel the pangs of poverty. Five years under treatment at home, in hospitals and in convalescence had stolen the little nest egg that had been hoped would some day provide the foundation for a home. The future appalled, and no wonder, for who can ever hope to stand for long against the ceaseless battering of ill health. No man is so constructed that he can resist forever. Such was the condition of one man who eventually came under my observation and direction in the search for better health.

The wife of this man happened to know an acquaintance of mine, who had unbounded faith in my abilities. Together they talked the situation over with me, which finally ended by my promise to see what I could do for him. He was only a young man as far as years were concerned; that is, he was only in his early thirties, thirty- two to be exact, but so much sickness had made him appear haggard and worn-out. Stomach trouble had necessitated an operation. I kept my appointment to talk over things, and the end of our conversation was that I carried hope into that home of trials. I talked to him something like this:

"Now look here, my friend, I know you are in a bad enough condition, and I realize your circumstances, but you have to remember that there is a beginning and an end for all things. There is a place and time for medicine, and a place and time for corrective exercise. You have long since arrived at the point where medicine finished and exercise should have begun. You have no kick against the

47

physicians; they have done their part. When they informed you that the cause of your stomach troubles was removed, it was practically all over for them. They gave you medicine to allay your sufferings and a specified diet for you to follow. Medicine will do a lot of things, but it will not rebuild weakened tissue. The trouble is you have relied too much upon medicine, and you failed to grasp the fact that your whole system had weakened through so much illness. Here is where exercise comes in. You do not have to look at me like that. I am not going to put a heavy weight in your hands and tell you to juggle it around, and at the same time practice Christian Science. It will be altogether different. You will find it a battle, but the chances are a hundred to one in your favor if you are game enough to struggle."

Well, we started the next day, and believe me or not, within three months from the date of our conversation he was helping around the house. Another four weeks saw him accepting a light position. Six! months after the day he commenced he was happily working at his old job, and within the year he was a picture of health. Not a Hercules, but much stronger than the average man. The sun was shining for him and the world appeared like an entirely new place to his wife and children.

This true story is not a miracle, or a near miracle. It is just common sense methods applied in the right place.

Too many people neglect their body in the first place, and it becomes a depository of dangerous elements that destroy tissue and lead to sickness. It is only natural that when a person becomes very sick, he should turn to his doctor and seek aid; but how many times do people have to listen to the physician say, "At some time or other you exposed yourself, and added neglect to exposure. This is the result." Then they realize that they are too late and have to face the music. Later the stage of convalescence is reached, usually after a harrowing experience, but it is the same story—neglect. The physician has performed his duty, and instead of the patient thinking a little for himself and profiting by the doctor's advice, he relies too much upon the doctor. Too frequently I hear the same story, "Oh, I've never been the same since that illness." Is there any wonder when they turn a deaf ear to nature? As the old scriptural phrase reads, "They have eyes but they see not."

The convalescent stage should be the commencement for remedial exercise. In making the following statement, I am not for one moment overlooking the fact that the physician is a very valuable man, and medicine one of our blessings; yet there are many ailments that can better be taken care of by exercise than by medicine, as my medical friends will agree.

"Stomach trouble, for instance. A common enough ailment, only too prevalent, but it is generally the result of a lack of body toning, bad eating, drinking alcoholic liquors and excessive smoking. Indigestion and hyperacidity are two of the worst, although the last is generally the cause of the first. Wrong functioning of the pancreas fails to absorb the fats, or break up the sugar and starch elements in the food. Although I have named the condition, incorrect functioning of the pancreas, I believe I would have been more correct if I had stated that wrong foods caused the pancreas to work overtime and have fagged it. The liver becomes sluggish as the digestion becomes poor. The biggest reason for the stomach disorders is lack of physical activity, that allows food to lie dormant too long in the stomach before it is dispelled into the channels of evacuation. This is one of the main causes of constipation, prolapsed stomach, and the unsightly protruding abdomen.

Now I want you to remember that the lining membranes of the stomach and bowels allow certain things from the food, like sugar molecules and little droplets of fat, to pass through just as water is passed through blotting paper. These particles enter into the veins, which are very numerous on the other side of the membranes. Consequently, you will readily realize the necessity of good digestion, and the natural requirements for these elements of nutrition to enter the blood stream. Food is absorbed in the blood very quickly, because the size of the absorbing surface is so large. It is actually claimed that the lining membranes of the stomach, the small and large intestines, taken together, have an area of twenty square feet. Somewhat more than the area of the entire outside of the body.

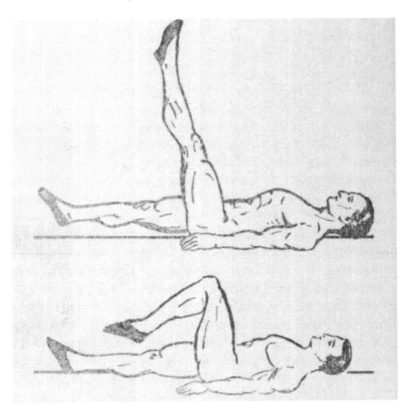

The more vigorous the daily vocation, the greater quantity of food is eaten, and the greater quantity of substance drawn into the blood stream, and also evacuation has more volume besides being more regular.

Your food is your energy, and it is a proposition entirely up to yourself whether you are going to use this energy or misuse it. The majority misuse it, hence the disorders. Now to correct these various ailments, I will select a few exercises that have a gentle persuasive effect upon the muscles, the organs of digestion, and the nervous system.

Take up your position with the hands placed upon the hips, feet spaced about six inches apart, just enough to keep the balance of the body comfortably. Bend from side to side in a slow, easy rhythmic movement. Let your breathing be regular and not forced in the least. Do not make the mistake of trying how many times you can do each exercise. About nine or ten times in each direction is enough with which to commence. In every case the individual should allow his physical condition to be his guide.

The next exercise should be taken up with the feet spaced much wider apart, with a light bar of ten or fifteen pounds lying across the broad of the back, each end grasped in the corresponding hand. From this position twist the body sideways from the waist, not the hips, in a spiral movement. As the body seems to be turned to its limit, the person should pull against the bar in order to obtain a little more twist. The reason the bar is allowed to lie across the shoulders, or broad of the back, instead of on the shoulders, is to gain more twist from the waist. It used to be that the exerciser would use the palms of each hand against the side of the chest, but my objection to this is that it causes a compression of the walls of the chest, interfering with both breathing and progress.

In all exercises where possible, I desire to see the person use some amount of weight; it helps to give a muscular resistance that cannot be supplied by the body only. Of course, if a person is in too weak a condition, that is different. Going back to the last exercise, I want to advise against allowing even the heels to leave the floor; that is why I suggest a waist movement against a hip movement. The feet must be kept flat on the floor.

For the third exercise I like to choose the one where the person lies upon the back on the floor, then slowly draws one knee up at a time to the body. In the second stage of progression, this exercise can be performed by drawing both knees, simultaneously, up to the body.

Then, turning over face downwards, so that the hands and toes only are resting upon the floor, with the arms locked at the elbows, and body straight upon its points of balance, we begin an exercise that is a little more vigorous. From the position described, draw the right knee up to the body, but allow the toes to rest on the floor. It is from here that the exercise is really commenced. Give a slight hop and straighten out the right leg, and at the same time pull the left knee up to the body. Do not hesitate, but keep both legs going one after the other. However, do not do it as though a race was being run; do it gently and always keep the hands on the floor.

These four exercises are quite enough with which to start, and as the conditions become improved and a greater degree of strength is acquired, more movements can be added and these can be eliminated for exercises of a more vigorous nature.

I know many have the idea that bending from the waist forwards and backwards are also good exercises. I agree, but the reason I have omitted them is because I want to say that people who are susceptible to vomiting from stomach disorders should not do them until after two or three weeks of practice with the other exercises. Where vomiting is not one of the troubles, the forward and backward bends are all right to use at the commencement.

These exercises are not as vigorous physically as those recommended for constipation and some other ailments. At the same time there is enough action to prepare the muscular toning for the exercises that follow in the various stages of progression. However, the circulatory organs are stimulated and the blood stream wonderfully nourished.

Constipation requires a somewhat more vigorous routine, due to the collection of feces that has clogged the intestinal passages. The exercises must be such that a continual massage is being brought to bear upon the intestines, at the same time that their natural functioning abilities are being repaired. Laxatives rob the channels of evacuation of their natural power. All along these passages are rings of muscles that contract and relax continually, and which gather and thrust the feces along the passages. As I have said, drugs interfere with the work of these muscles by relieving them of their natural duty, and the trouble is that the muscles deteriorate with non-use. When the body has become used to the effect of the drugs, which it does in time, the person faces a serious proposition.

However, I have known of many chronic cases of constipation effectively cured by exercise. The muscles of the abdomen are naturally equipped to aid the thousands of ring muscles that are part of the intestines.

Body builders have made the expression habitual, when describing the abdominal muscles, as having a washboard appearance. They have more than a washboard appearance; they have the washboard effect, continually massaging the intestines in order to prevent solidification of feces and stimulate evacuation; but we never see a victim of this ailment with a well developed set of abdominal muscles. In most cases the waistline is large, sagging, and fat. The muscles have lost their elasticity, and the armor of muscle protection is gone. A victim can wear all the body belt sup-porters he likes, but nothing like that will give back life to the deteriorated muscular tissue.

In a chronic case, I generally advise a few days fast, in order to give the stomach a rest. As a matter of fact, a short fast is sometimes advisable with stomach trouble, but not in all cases. A person should always seek advice on this before going ahead on his own initiative.

Since the working powers of the muscles have gone, we are obliged to devise exercises that will perform these duties as much as possible, and at the same time coax these muscles back into vigorous existence and build them up. The most commonly known exercise for the abdomen is the "sit-up." In this exercise the person lies full length on the back upon the floor, with some heavy object across the feet to hold the legs down as the sit-up is made.

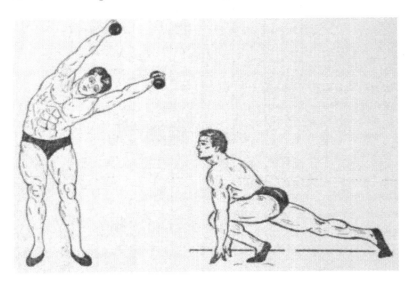

This is performed by either folding the arms upon the chest or locking the hands behind the neck. From the prone position the exerciser rises to the sit-up position, and then lowers the body back, repeating the movement a number of times. Personally, I do not like the exercise from a curative point of view, in fact, not for a beginner. My objection is based upon the fact that beginners, who are not seeking curative aid, are seldom able to perform the movement correctly. They invariably come up with a snap, which is wrong. Others cannot do it at all. A very few can. The movement should be done slowly in both raising and lowering the body, so that the muscles receive full play and give the desired effect upon the intestines. I prefer this exercise for a more advanced stage of muscle building. In its place I advocate sitting upon the floor with the feet under some object, back straight, and the arms folded behind the back, leaning at the slightest possible angle backwards. From this position twist the body from side to side as much as possible with a slow movement. After this, lie flat upon the floor on the back, then place the hands on the floor and raise the body until the arms are straight and only the hands and heels are resting on the floor. Keep the body free from any bend. Now raise one leg straight as high as you can. Keep the legs moving thus, one after the other. Then you can practice drawing the knees up to the body alternately. Both exercises are good.

In the more advanced exercises, I find that raising the body onto the shoulders, from the prone position, with the hands pressed upon the hips, and the elbows on the floor as a means of support, is a very good body reducer and aid for constipation. From this position the legs should be worked up and down in a movement similar to pedaling a bicycle. This exercise can be followed, by another exercise from the prone position. Lie flat upon the back and place the hands under the hips, then raise one leg upwards in a circular movement towards the head. As the leg is lowered, the heel should not be allowed to touch the floor; then raise the other leg. Keep the legs straight, raising and lowering in a slow rhythmic movement. After this, the same position can be adopted, and both legs raised together.

As a further aid a good massage of the abdominal muscles will help considerably.

The beauty of the last two exercises is that they develop the muscles of the abdomen from the lower extremities of the abdomen upwards. This part of the abdomen is of the most importance. From the line of the navel down into the groin, the fourth twin muscle of the abdomen begins and ends. It is in this region that the appendix becomes affected, and hernia is made possible or impossible, according to the state of development in which the muscles are. I have seen many body culturists who could show a nice upper abdominal display, but were sadly neglectful of the lower part. That is another fault of the "sit-up." It develops mostly the abdominals from the chest to the navel, and the last pair of muscles which are long and wedge shaped are almost passed over. The exercise where one and both legs are raised while lying on the back in the prone position is the best, as it gets them all. Better progression can be made upon this exercise, by increasing the resistance by hooking a light kettle bell over each foot.

These last two exercises, and the shoulder stand, or bicycle tread, are effective in strengthening the lower torso, and should be among the exercises used by those who feel that they have a tendency to rupture. The external oblique muscles should be specialized upon in hernia tendencies. I have actually known of several cases of hernia cured by these and other exercises.

Hernia is the result of weak musculature. The muscles of the body are our anatomical protectors, and if we neglect them we are trifling with our lives equally as much as the soldier who forgets his rifle.

An exercise that I like very much for strengthening the external oblique muscles is practiced by taking a fairly light dumb-bell in each hand, of about fifteen pounds each, then raise them to arms' length overhead, and stand with the feet set firmly apart. Look up at the dumb-bells and lean over sideways as far as you can, then straighten up and lean over to the other side. Keep up the movement, and you will find that the weights held overhead will cause a great leverage from the external oblique muscles in order to bring the body back to the erect position. Then again, the dumb-bells are so light that the arms will not tire before the side muscles get their workout, and the overhead principle provides a fine leverage upon which the exercise can be made progressively more difficult.

Do not practice the "sit-up" or the leaning forward exercise with a weight held behind the neck, if you feel the tissue of the groin to be weak. In fact, do not perform any exercises that have a bearing down tendency upon the abdomen. Exercises performed upside down are always good and can be safely practiced.

Perhaps the condition of nervousness is another of the most common ailments that; often makes life seem unbearable. A nervous person may not be too sick to work, but he finishes the day ragged, and always on edge. This condition, more than any other, is a lack of body toning. It is invariably a condition of the nerve cells that have been deprived of the necessary amount of nutriment in proportion to nerve expenditure. Among people whose vocation involves more mental effort than physical, are found the largest number of sufferers. The muscles of the body lie under the skin practically useless, expending none of their surplus energy, and conserving none. Your batteries are running on their own reserve, and that cannot last. What we put out must be accounted for. Nature demands some form of recuperation, and that is only obtained from physical stimulus. Insomnia is one of the big evils resultant upon nervousness. Even the hours nature has set on one side for recuperation and conservation are stolen by this fiend. But it is a condition that has to be decided by the individual. It is not a condition which has to be put up with, or that cannot be overcome. Exercise will solve the problem.

A number of years ago, one of my clients, who was one of the biggest business men in America, was a nervous wreck, and on two occasions I was informed he had tried to end his life. Everything, apparently, had been done. The best experts in one thing and another had failed. Two of our foremost physical instructors had failed, and also an imported expert from Europe. I was later approached, and when I had my first interview with this millionaire, he frankly told me that he did not believe anyone could help him. I talked to him, and he placed his confidence in me, and inside of three months I had a new man.

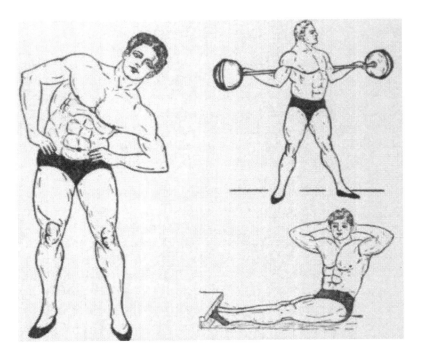

According to our tests he had improved 230 per cent, and he showed his gratitude to me in many ways. I applied psychology with exercise in this case and won. I try to apply psychology with every person I handle. In the thousands whom I have handled, I have learned a lot in applying it. I study them, place myself in their shoes, and figure out what I would do in the ignorance of facts. Ultimately I see their problems, and my knowledge and experience on health and body building have successfully helped me to bridge the gap and restore all who were willing to help me, help them.

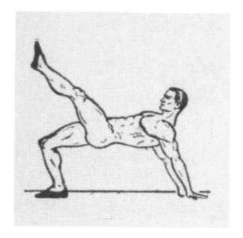

CHAPTER V
BUILDING A MIGHTY CHEST

The first thing about Henry Steinborn that inspired me was his magnificent chest. Although the rest of his proportions were splendidly formed, yet his chest appealed to me as one of the most magnificent I had ever seen. The width, the depth and the unusual prominence, all gave forcible evidence of terrific concealed power. Unlike many other large chests I have seen, the chest of Steinborn begins to rise from the throat with a powerful surge that falls squarely over the entire thorax. It looks like a big square box with the edges rounded, so massive is its construction. A great many athletes rely upon the development of the latissimus dorsi; for their largest chest measurement, which does not correctly explain the actual size of the chest. I suppose most of you know what I mean, but for the benefit of those who are not so familiar with the influence of the latissimus dorsi muscles upon the chest, I will explain that many athletes give their expanded chest measurement as a proof of its size and in order to make it appear larger than it really is, they flex the latissimus dorsi which causes these muscles to spread out, giving the upper body a fanlike appearance. Any fairly well developed body culturist can increase the tape measurement at least two inches by performing this muscular movement. I have actually known two cases where the measure showed an eight inch increase by flexing these muscles after the chest had been expanded to its limit, but you can plainly see that it is not a true indication of chest size. The normal chest measurement is the honest indication of what your chest is. If you were to tell me that your normal chest measured thirty-six inches, but it was forty inches expanded, it would be the first measurement which would guide me in estimating the qualifications of your thorax. It is the space that is naturally allotted to your heart and lungs in the ordinary circumstance that counts most. What space can be supplied in one single movement of expansion, is only a minor consideration in chest power.

Actually, the more powerfully constructed is the chest, the less expansion it has. A person who suffers from asthma, bronchitis, and tuberculosis has much greater chest expansion than the athlete with the best built chest. Struggling for breath causes the lungs to become abnormal in expansion, although the reaction from this is that the walls of the chest cave in, and the muscle deteriorates so that normally the chest is a sorrowful sight. In this condition, the lungs become elongated by the abnormal relaxation of the rib box, and the sternum of the chest become hollow. All this means that ordinarily the breathing space is very limited, and the supply of oxygen drawn into the respiratory organs is all too insufficient to combat the amount of carbon dioxide that saturates the life chambers of the lungs.

A great deal of our success in body building relies upon the amount of success that is reached in developing a powerful chest. There is no doubt that we all admire a well built chest, and we all want to possess one with all its attendant qualities, without which, the chest becomes a sepulcher. At one time there was an awful fad among young men to appear as though they had a finely built chest, which brought about the forced chest condition, and a very lamentable condition at that. A young man was taught to be constantly conscious of his chest, and walk with it thrust out, and to further aid the condition, they had their clothes made to suit the occasion. It was very amusing to see a man of very slim stature wearing a suit cut full at the chest and the shoulders padded, and from the center was sticking a scrawny pipe stem neck. This method of walking with the chest forced out was an old army habit which developed the "puffed chest" condition, so termed by army medical men. It had a very serious effect upon the heart, and when this was found out, the forced attitude was discouraged. I tried it, like everyone else, but it gave me such pain that I quickly gave it up. I was very young at that time, but I was fortunate in receiving advice from a very well informed instructor, who taught me the difference between holding the shoulders back and thrusting the chest out.

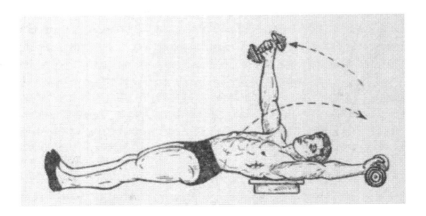

You know you can't go after chest growth like you can that of. any other part of the body,—there are too many things to take into consideration, including the heart, lungs, the structure of the chest and its muscular coating. The exercises must be such that no organic stress is evinced, and apart from exercising to increase the chest size, adequate consideration must be given to the increase of muscular tissue in order to hold the gains, and thus provide the natural method of retaining the chest size obtained from exercise.

Did it ever occur to you how it is possible for the chest to increase its size, when ordinarily the average person figures the construction of the chest is all bone? "How can you stretch bone?" has been the unanswerable question in many minds. Hundreds have asked me that question, and I have even had people take the other side and ask "Now, if it is possible to increase the chest, which is a mass of bones, why can't we stretch our back bone, our thigh and calf bones, so that a very short person can be made much taller?" Well, offhand there would seem to be no logical reason why this could not be done, looking at the question in the light they do. But, we know that neither is correct. We have to delve into anatomy to understand it correctly. I hope you do not get tired reading the various anatomical explanations. I know they sound rather dry, but the only way to understand whether the explanatory advice is correct, is to analyze the construction of what we have in mind. Our subjects have to be educational as well as instructive, so we must tackle the chest in this manner.

The thorax, as a whole, commences at the throat and extends downwards to where the abdomen commences. It is composed of twelve pair of ribs that appear to have a barrel shape formation. All these ribs have a double connection with the exception of the last two pair, which are known as the floating ribs and are free in the muscles of the flank. The first seven pair articulate with the sternum, more commonly known as the breast bone, by means of their cartilaginous attachment. You must remember that each of the ribs are attached to the spine with a cartilage, but the first five are directly fastened to the breast bone, and the sixth and seventh join together and then divide to be separately attached at the base of the sternum. These seven pair of ribs are termed the true ribs, and as the other five are not attached to the sternum in the same manner, they are called the false ribs. The first three of the last five ribs, that would be the eighth, ninth and tenth, are united by their cartilage to the cartilage of the seventh rib. The remaining two are, as I have previously stated, the floating ribs, and have only one attachment, which is on the spine. These cartilages are all termed costal cartilages, which means rib attachments.

Now the sternum, or breast bone, is divided into three sections. The first rib is fastened to the first section and the second rib is attached at the joint, midway of the first and second section. The second section of the frontal bone is the largest, and the one to which all the other costal cartilages are attached. The third part is very small, being tail-like in fashion. The word sternum means, "connection with" which explains the true nature of the breast bone as a part that connects the costal cartilages. Apart from the rib attachments, the pectoral, or breast muscles have an origination here, and the sternum helps to support the clavicle.

Now, let us go back and see how it is we can increase the chest size by a natural process. In order to do this, we must make our exercises co-ordinate with the natural construction of the chest formation. Nothing must have a false origination, or influence, so we must commence with an analysis of the information we have on hand. When we raise up the chest, not necessarily expand it, the upheaval hinges upon that first dividing place of the sternum bone, and when we expand the chest, it is the muscular action without and the volume of air inhaled, that together cause the ribs to be spread apart by this action. The cartilages stretch in order to make this possible. Therefore, to make the chest naturally increase, and stay so, the muscles that surround the chest must be exercised in such a manner that they not only spread the rib sector, but accumulate the muscular tissue to such proportion that they will retain the growth. Exercises that simply spread or expand the chest, as is the case with all free movements, do not mean a thing. Undoubtedly they give a greater expansion, but that means nothing, as the heart and lungs do not acquire any greater space for natural inspiration. The most important muscles of the chest are the pectorals, and the serratus magnus, and as these muscles acquire growth, so do the cartilages of the ribs become longer, thicker and more secure in their attachment. As this process takes place, the chest becomes deeper, higher and more square. The muscular coating is heavier and more protective. These muscles are the real agencies of chest growth, and since we have made ourselves fully familiar with the rib construction and articulation to such an extent, that we know the course nature takes in promoting chest growth, we will pass on and study the whys and wherefores of these muscular agencies, so every chest builder can obtain the results that will overcome all his chest difficulties.

Hollow chests, by reason of their sunken appearance, worry a person the most, but when a chest has caved in, it is easy to see that the walls of the chest have fallen in also. But this condition is not quite as noticeable. Yet, in all such cases, it will be found that the breast muscles are very undeveloped. The pectorals are so named for they are armor plates, or covers. Like plates of armor they cover the entire upper part of the chest. They are divided in two sections on each side, into minor and major muscles. The origination of the major muscle is upon the sternum bone, and finally becomes attached in the biceptal groove of the humerus bone, upon which the biceps of the arm is lodged. The end of this muscle tapers off into a very strong flat tendon, that seems to disappear under the deltoid muscle on its way to insertion in the humerus. The minor pectoral lies somewhat underneath, and is attached upon the breast bone in the region of the third, fourth and fifth rib, and is also inserted by a flat tendon, but into the scapula or shoulder blade.

As I explain all this, my mind goes back to the days when all this material was more or less of a mystery to me.

I used to read anatomical books, but I was completely swamped by those long technical names that were so devoid of understanding to the layman. Maybe it is this reason why I take length, and perhaps more than the necessary care, to explain it all to you in an understanding way, free of all technical phrases. A simple analysis enables you to immediately visualize where these muscles originate and become inserted, then you are better able to realize how they operate. The action of the pectoral major is such that it draws the arm forward and inward, and is termed an accessory muscle of forced inspiration. By this I mean the muscle is an aid to stimulate the breathing. By bringing the arms forward the chest is contracted, and by spreading the arms which includes the help of the serratus magnus, the chest becomes expanded and thus helps the lungs to inhale and exhale. Then we must figure that any movement that brings the arms forward and inward, is the best to promote the development of the breast muscles. Some very good exercises come to my mind immediately, which I know you can practice with profit.

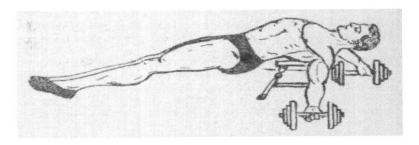

The first is an old exercise of mine that I practiced ever since I was a youngster, and which I always enjoyed. Take your position standing erect. The feet can be placed any way to suit yourself, as they do not count in this exercise. Hold a light dumb-bell in each hand, then breathe in gently and at the same time begin to cross the arms across the chest, just as far as you possibly can. The arms must be kept straight, and no deflation of the chest take place before the arms begin to travel back to their original position at the side. As a form of variation, it is a good idea to allow the left arm to cross under the right arm, and then on the repeat, allow the right arm to cross under the left. Keep the chest held high, and do not bend the arms the least bit, and I will guarantee that your breast muscles will receive vigorous play.

Another fine exercise performed from the erect position with a pair of dumb-bells, is as follows: From the sides you simply raise one bell until it is held straight out in front on a level with the shoulder; as the arm descends, raise the other, but see that the dumb bell is held end ways with the floor, in each hand. This same movement can be practiced by holding a very light bar bell, but it must be light. With a heavier poundage, I use this exercise for a very important forearm muscle developer which I will explain in its proper place.

The pectoral minor operates in a slightly different manner, inasmuch as they are muscles of depression, as well as being very important in elevating the chest when the shoulder blades are drawn back. Without inflating the chest just draw the shoulder blades together, and you will feel the pull from these muscles and the chest will rise. Also, while the arms are hanging by the sides, clench the fists and without bending the body, thrust downwards and you will feel the pectorals contract as you do so. Therefore, you can see if you hold a fairly heavy dumb-bell in each hand, by pressing downwards, the Weight of the dumb-bells will aid you and give greater contraction to the muscles.

Some exercise fans find it difficult to always have their outfit with them, and feel they would like to keep up the good work. I never like to see them have to lay off, if it can be prevented in any way, so for their benefit, I would advise them to practice the following exercises without weights. Clasp the hands upon the chest, and without allowing the body to be twisted in the least from the waist, force the left hand across the chest with the right hand, and at the same time resist with the left hand, until the right arm is straightened out across the chest. Then force the right arm back with the left, applying the same form of resistance. However, always bear in mind to keep the hands close to the chest throughout the exercise. Then, practice the regular floor dip which is an exercise common to all. I might say that the first group of exercises can be practiced to an advantage when the use of weights is not possible.

Some athletes develop beautiful breast muscles, the finest of which I know are those that adorn the chest of Andrew Passanant. J. Trullio also has fine breast muscles. However, this training can be overdone. If other parts of the body are not taken care of equally, the breast muscles will draw the shoulders forward. Wrestlers usually have very large breast muscles from constantly hugging their opponents, therefore wrestling can be practiced to an advantage for pectoral development.

Now let us consider the serratus magnus muscles for a while. I do not believe my readers are quite as familiar with these muscles as they are with the pectorals. In fact, I have been surprised at the number of letters I have received asking me where these muscles are located, and just what they do.

The prominence of these muscles has given rise to some amusing comments. It is not unusual to hear a person exclaim, after studying a photo of chest development, "Look how his ribs show." Well, I must admit that to the uninitiated, they do give that impression, but what is actually prominent, is the serratus magnus muscles. These muscles are even more powerful in inspiration than the pectorals. They have their insertion on the scapula bone or shoulder blade, and arise from the space of nine ribs. From their insertion, they separate or become, as their name implies, serrated, which in another way means to acquire a saw tooth formation. When viewed upon a well developed chest, they have the appearance of spread fingers. In fact, as you will later see, the hand and its fingers give a fine interpretation of how these muscles function. Each of these nine serrated points, are lodged upon nine of the ribs, all in different lengths. Most of this great muscle covers the intercostal spaces at the back, and partly on the sides, before they reach their costal, or rib attachment. (By inter- costal, I mean the spaces between the ribs.) Now here is something I want you to remember, so you will better understand the threefold action of this muscle. It is because the insertion of the serratus magnus is threefold upon the scapula, that it is so powerful in its movements of inspiration. Any movement that gives action in all positions that are vertical, horizontal and rotary, belongs partly to the serratus. For instance, raise your arms overhead, then from the shoulder stretch them out level with the shoulders. After this, slowly rotate the arm in a circular movement, and in all these movements you will feel "pulls" that have a varying effect upon the chest. In all such actions the serratus magnus operates. You will also gather the idea that the back muscles are going to get a lot of help out of this, which is true. A man with a good chest invariably has good back muscles. Bar bell users always display the best developed serratus magnus muscles, and also all they who follow weight lifting as a sport, by reason of lifting heavy weights overhead. As these muscles contract, they bring about a pulling and an uplifting action upon the chest which causes the saw tooth attachments to spread the walls of the chest, by stretching the costal cartilages. If you close your hand and then open it, stretching the fingers, and bend the hand upon the wrist you will get a similar movement of what takes place, as the scapula is moved by the arm, compelling a serratus movement.

I have a few more exercises in mind, which I believe are the very best for stimulating the increase in chest size and muscular growth. At the same time, I want to warn you against certain others which some people will insist upon doing despite the detrimental effects.

The two arm pull over has been advocated very strongly during the last few years, although I am not one who insisted on its practice as the best thing, because I know this exercise is fraught with a condition, after a certain point is reached, that does more harm than good. I know the exercise is a good one, but only up to a certain point, then again, I know other exercises which are much better, and have not the attendant danger of the two arm pull over. This last named exercise was originally taught in the following manner.

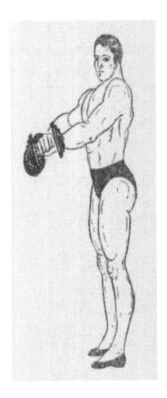

The pupil would lie flat upon the floor with a light bar bell lying across the thighs, grasped with both hands, the arms of which would be straight. From this position the weight would be raised in a half circular movement, until it rested upon the floor at arms' length behind the head. All the time the arms are kept straight, and the back kept as flat as possible upon the floor. The bar bell would be brought back to the original position in the same half circular movement. Later, this exercise was changed. No doubt because many complained that when they had reached a certain weight, they were not able to move the bell off their thighs, and yet the weight appeared to be so light as to have not the sufficient pull upon the chest. In order to give greater chest action, the movement was made quarter circular. The starting place for the bell this time, was at arms' length over the face and lowered to arms' length at the back of the head. The trouble was that it gave too much chest action. Exercise fans who were eager to build a big chest began to crowd on the weight; the result was that a great depression of the diaphragm took place, and the space became too congested which began to crowd the heart. I strongly disapprove of any exercise that will cause a protracted isolation of the diaphragm. It is not natural. Many who have practiced this, complained to me of how their heart would palpitate after. Such is always the case. They found the amount of weight easy to handle until the weight was about six inches off the floor, lowering and raising the weight. When these points were reached, the deltoid action became similar to a hold out in front. A position where little weight can be handled. Many of them develop kinks in the deltoid for the same reason. Remember, it is a good exercise as long as you do not exceed twenty-five pounds, if you are a light man. Fifty pounds is enough for any man. Of the two methods of performing this exercise, I prefer the first, because the exerciser is restricted with weight at a position where no harm possibly can occur. A much better exercise is to take up the position upon the floor with the back between the shoulders resting upon the seat of a low stool, and the heels on the floor. Take in each hand a ten pound dumb-bell, and hold at arms' length over the face.

From this position begin to breathe in and lower the bells down sideways, as low as your shoulders will permit. While keeping the arms straight return to the original position. About ten counts is enough to start on and work up to twenty movements as the limit, then use heavier dumb-bells and start out with ten counts again.

From this same position, on the stool, another exercise can be done that is good. Instead of lowering the arms outwards as before, lower them in opposite directions parallel with the body. That is, the left arm would travel to arms' length behind the head, and the right to arms' length by the side. Each arm working in this manner with the same amount of weight and conditions governing it as in the last exercise will help to build for you a mighty chest of which you can be proud.

CHAPTER VI
IS THERE SUCH A THING AS BONE STRENGTH?

I know that the mere suggestion that bones are capable of demonstrating strength would be accepted by many people with a doubtful mind. The majority firmly believe that the bones are simply props and connections by which the body is held together. Apart from that, their use in our existence is believed to be minor as compared with the other organs of the body. Of course, it is partly true that the bones exist for that reason, but there are many other important uses for this structure, to which my readers may never have given thought. As a matter of fact, I do not ever remember seeing where the bones were discussed in the light that our title brings before us. Some writers who take a joy in decrying strength feats as being all faked, like to dwell upon feats where terrific poundages are held upon the body as an illustration of their claims. They call it all fake in their ignorance, and for comparison they will make a statement something like this: "There was Saxon. He claimed to be the strongest man in the world, and the best he ever raised was four hundred forty-eight pounds overhead with two hands. Then, there is that fellow Strongfort, who claims the same title, because he has held up an automobile that weighs about two tons. Just look at the difference in weight, which goes to show neither is right." You know this is the way they talk, and the very fact that they talk like this is positive proof of how little they know about what they say. Of course, the difference in poundage is staggering if you want to look at it that way, but knowledge of the body undeniably informs us that there can be no comparison between the two feats. Both are actual feats of strength, but just as widely separated as the difference between a sprint racer and a five mile run. In the case under discussion, one is strength of muscle, and the other is strength of bone.

Let us take a little lesson in their structure and find the truth for ourselves in the wonders of bone formation. Instead of being just props for the mass of muscles to surround, we find that the bones are the levers of the bodies, fulfilling their duties as nature required, just as the muscles act as the motors, and the ligaments as the pulleys. They all work together. Just take a derrick for example, and you have the analysis pat. The engine is the power behind the chain that hoists, and the beam is the instrument of leverage.

The structure of the bone itself is a dense form of connective tissue, impregnated with inorganic matter, chiefly calcium phosphate, to which its hardness and rigidity is due. In other words, the bones are a cartilagus formation, and the appearance of the life chemical, calcium phosphate, is what causes the bones to ossify or harden. Not all the bones in the body acquire the state of ossification as found in the bones in the arms, thighs, hips and the scapula. Take for instance the ribs, sternum and clavicle. While they are much smaller than the bones mentioned, yet because they retain their cartilagus condition in a less concrete form, for natural reasons, they are capable of bending to a greater degree than other bones before they will break. Altogether, there are two hundred and six bones in the body, counting the three parts of the sternum bone as just one. It is in the marrow of our bones that the tiny red corpuscles are born. These corpuscles are as important to our existence as the heart itself, as they form the major part of the blood stream and give this life flowing stream its color. Strange as it may seem, like the tissue of our muscles, these little corpuscles wear out after a few weeks, and new corpuscles from the bone marrow take their place and live their short life, and so on. Of course, you understand without my explanation how these corpuscles get into the bloodstream, by being injected through the porous structure of the bone. Now this little fact alone will give you some idea of bone formation. You cannot help but see right away that the healthier a person is, the better bone structure he is going to have. A person who is anemic can put the cause down to the fact that the supply of red corpuscles are not being manufactured in sufficient quantities to supply the need which can all be traced to lack of body toning in the first place. The ultimate resistance of the bones will always depend upon the general condition of the body. It is a positive fact that healthy bones are bound to have healthy strong attachments. These fleshy attachments will cleave to the bones more securely. Perhaps this is best borne out by the relative condition of the bones in one who has trained his body and he who has not. Medical statistics prove that the laboring man has construction ally thicker bones than the clerical worker.

The answer to this is a purely natural one. It works out just the same as the muscular condition, as explained in the chapter, "Defining the Mystery of Strength." If the clerical man had to change his occupation for one that involved manual labor, a bone thickening process would take place, along with the change in musculature. Of course, the change is not so noticeable and never so radical as is often seen in the muscular change. Nevertheless, the bones do not have to increase their thickness very much to be able to withstand a resistance that altogether is equal to one thousand pounds. Take a young athlete who has started bar bell training, and test him on his supporting ability as well as his muscular strength. Inside of a month his supporting abilities will have gone up tremendously in comparison with his regular lifting tests. At the same time, the increase in bone size could hardly be registered, but just the same a great change has taken place. The bones have acquired a greater resistance from the healthier condition of the body.

It really is surprising to notice the peculiar conception that the ordinary individual has about the body, which, of course, includes the bony framework. I have heard many people who had, at some time in their life, been so unfortunate as to break a limb, say that they were afraid to make a lift for fear they would break that member again. They firmly believe that the bone is weaker where it was broken, and they will shrink from making what was formerly a very ordinary lift. When you stop to consider the plea, you will find it a natural misunderstanding among laymen. Actually, the bone is stronger after the injury than it was before. That is providing the bone has been set right at the time. Under X-ray examination, the bone will be found much thicker at the broken part than elsewhere. The knitting process of the bone when healing is much like a weld upon iron where the smith generally leaves it slightly thicker. A smith will tell you that the iron will always break elsewhere, providing he made a good weld. So it is with the bone. It is a matter of interest to know that pugilists of the bare fist age were known to break their arms on purpose, so that shock from hard striking would be better absorbed. The famous prize fighter, Tom Sayers, was only a light man, but his great hitting powers enabled him to knock out much bigger opponents than himself. Both his arms had been frequently broken—mostly in fights—and many boxing followers of the present time, who do not know of that former practice, and wonder how that little man could stand up and batter big men and stand it, as he did in his memorable battle with Hennan, should remember that Sayers attributed it to his thickened bones caused by the breaks. They also used to pickle their hands in brine to toughen them and make them so hard that the hand was less inclined to be knocked out of joint or broken.

One of our star wrestlers, with whom I am very familiar, used to complain about his left wrist being weak. He was always afraid of it. During a contest he was thrown off the mat and landed with such impact upon his hands and knees, that his left wrist was broken. About a year or so after the accident I was talking to him, and he remarked how singular it was, but since the accident, his left wrist was the stronger and how he used it the most in clinching his locks. Nothing singular about it; just nature showing how well it does a job. Of course I do not want you to go out and break an arm, or anything like that. I am just bringing these conditions forward as an example of how the bone structure works, and to explain that people who have sustained a broken arm or leg should not worry. A broken hip, or joint, is entirely different. The former control is seldom acquired afterwards.

Now to get back to the actual strength of bones as supplied to us in feats of strength, let me say that there is a world of difference in lifting weight, holding weights, and supporting feats of strength. In lifting a weight overhead, one just has their muscular power operating. While muscular strength has greater motive power, yet it has no rigid control over gravity, or the weight, until it is at the shoulders or at arms' length overhead. Greater weight can be held at the shoulders and at arms' length overhead than can be actually lifted, simply because the locking process of the elbows, shoulders and knees provide greater sustaining power. It is the spine in the lumbar region, or the small of the back, that gives way first in holding a weight aloft. Simply because in that region there is no other supporting bone structure than the spine itself, and the natural curve in the spine does not provide a perfect perpendicular resistance.

Supporting feats are performed in positions that generally involve the legs, hips and arms, and in some instances, to a certain extent, the back. But never is the weight actually lifted. It is always supported; and the positions in which the athlete places himself are such, that the greatest aid is given to the bony structure, to enable the

77

performer to support the most weight and thereby appear more spectacular and astounding. As we go along explaining this feature you will see that all the weight is borne upon the bones with a perpendicular pressure. In such a manner, the bones are capable of greater resistance, than when the resistance is thrown upon them laterally.

A feat of supporting strength that is commonly performed is the one known as "the tomb of Hercules." The athlete takes up his position with the hands and feet only upon the floor, and the face looking upwards. The hands are turned back along a line parallel with the body which gives a better arm lock in the elbows. The body is held up fairly well, but not so high as to have the body level with the line of the knees and the shoulders. The arms and legs from the foot to the knee must be perpendicular so that no lateral pressure is suggested. Then a platform is placed on the body so that it has four points of rest, both knees and the shoulders. A number of men are then seated upon the board, which is supported by the athlete for a few seconds. Some athletes make this stunt more spectacular by supporting a whole orchestra while it plays, and others allow an automobile to run over a trestle supported in this manner. In this latter feat, the machine is only supported a bare fraction of a second, and the fact that the machine is moving across distributes the weight so that actually the entire weight of the machine is not supported all at one time by the body. But enough weight is supported to make the act very dangerous. If I remember rightly, Monte Saldo, an English athlete, was one of the first to introduce this stunt. Then came Strongfort. The last man to perform this feat within the last few years was Wilfred Cabana, of Montreal, but he sustained some serious accidents from it, and has discarded it since, so I understand. Due to the fact that the machine is moving all the time, I do not consider this as great a test of bone strength, as the feat where a man supports an orchestra of ten or twelve men.

The Englishman, Appelton, was very good at this stunt, and claims to have supported two thousand four hundred and ninety- two pounds, but I am sure, good though this support is, men like Travis, who by the way used to support a carousel in this manner,—Giroux, Steinborn and particularly Moerke would easily pass that mark.

In all these feats there is a certain amount of muscular force required. If the arm triceps are not strong, the elbows will unlock under the pressure, just the same as the feet slip away if the biceps of the thighs are not strong enough.

Saxon was great at all this stuff, but his specialty supporting stunt lay in a more difficult performance, in which the major portion of the weight was supported by the legs. For this feat he would lie on his back and place a bar bell that weighed 267 pounds on the soles of his feet, and over the toes of each foot he hung a kettle bell that weighed 100 pounds each; then his partners would place six men on the bar bell. This done, Saxon pulled a bar bell over his face from the back of his head and raised it to arms' length. On each end of this bell, each of his partners sat. What the total weight was I do not remember ever hearing, but assuming that the six men on the feet averaged 150 pounds each, and they would be likely to average more, as Saxon always got the heaviest men possible, the total weight on the feet alone would be 1307 pounds. This is a terrific feat when you consider that this mass of weight had to be balanced as well as supported; and the control required in itself is a great tax on strength. The slightest bending of the knees, and the results would be disastrous. One of the most astounding supporting feats of all times was their stunt billed as the "Brooklands on Legs." Arthur Saxon and one of his younger brothers would lie on their back under a huge wooden trestle, and with their feet support the whole affair, while a loaded automobile ran over the trestle. In this act, they were not able to hold the legs entirely straight, that is the knees were bent a little. By pressing with the hands against the knees, a bracing support was given, which made up, to a certain extent, for the bending of the knees. But they did it once too often. Something went wrong, and the whole thing came down on them. They were both badly injured, and the younger brother refused to have anything to do with it afterwards. It was estimated that the whole load weighed six thousand five hundred pounds. In our time, those two famous Germans, Herman Gorner and Karl Moerke, have proven themselves great at supporting feats, as well as other feats that call for great muscular strength. Gorner has actually supported the terrific weight of twenty men sitting on a plank that rested on his feet, with straight legs, a total weight of four thousand pounds. This[1] is the greatest weight, supported in that manner, I ever heard of. However, Gorner is an extraordinary being.

I saw a picture of Moerke taken over in Hoboken, New York, where he was lying upon his back, and with his leg strength, raised and supported the front end of the Hoboken Fire Engine. In another feat, a-la Saxon, Moerke eclipsed the great Arthur's poundage by supporting about fifteen hundred pounds on the feet only. But this squat German, is naturally adapted to these trials. His legs are short, and carry a thigh measurement of twenty- eight and a half inches and calf of seventeen and a half inches. Then on the other hand, he is not a large boned man, which brings to our mind the thought that after all, there may be the same difference in bone structure as in muscle tissue. However, I am quite satisfied that bone strength exists. It has a limit to its possibilities just the same as muscular strength. Take, for instance, the recent accident to Henry Steinborn. He tried to do the "Brooklands on Legs," all alone. He found the poundage more than he could handle and broke a leg. My memory goes back to Rudolph Klar who used to regularly hold anywhere from eight to ten men supported on his feet. One day he tried eighteen men and the resistance proved too much, and he broke his legs.

There are various methods of supporting weights, and while we are at it, we might as well take them all in consideration. One of the other feats, is to hold a bar bell across the shoulders behind the neck, and allow a number of men to hang on each side. Saxon, nightly in his act, would hold a bar bell of 232 pounds across his shoulders and allow four men to swing on at each side, a total weight of over fourteen hundred pounds. Some athletes try to walk with this burden, and in so doing they march sideways instead of forwards, so that no bend in the knees takes place; if it does, the lifter is not able to sustain the weight.

One of the popular feats of years ago was a hip lift in harness. The lifter had a leather attachment around his hips, and standing high upon a perch he would pile a group of people on a platform underneath. This done, he would hitch his hip harness with a hook, onto the apparatus below, and by pressing with the hands on a rail that ran at each side of the perch, begin the feat. The combined hip and arm pressure raises the platform with its human load just high enough to swing clear of its rest and that was just high enough for him to lock his knees. Then the rest was easy. Some of them have the weight lowered down gradually, instead of raising it, and consequently more weight is handled. It is almost impossible to break the hips from such resistance, as the pelvis bone forms a natural arch. The only thing that can happen is for the pressure to unlock the knees.

By lying upon the back, and drawing up the knees until they are at right angles with the body, and then having the legs, from the knees to the ankle, held at right angles with the thighs so that the legs and body presents a letter Z, an athlete places himself in a position where he can support a lot of weight. All that is required is a board placed across the top of the knees so that a downward pressure is brought upon the thigh bone into the hip. A number of men can easily be supported thus, and the feat always looks better if the athlete pulls over a bar bell with his hands and raises it to straight arms, and then allows a man to sit on each end.

The reason why so much weight can be lifted in the back and the harness lift, is because the body is placed in such a position that the muscles are capable of applying their greatest motive power. The weight is only lifted an inch or two, and the weight is so distributed upon the legs, back and arms, in a back lift, and the hips and legs in a harness lift, that the weight is not hard to control. The athlete is in a very unique position to hold his load.

It is not everybody who can perform these stupendous supporting feats. It takes a trained athlete, a man who has cultivated his body, and given it the best of care during his life time. It is wrong to say that a support is not a feat of strength. A support of a thousand pounds in one of these feats has its place in the annals of strength, just the same as the raising of a bar bell of three hundred pounds overhead. The only difference is that one is bone strength and the other is muscular strength. The only wrong thing about it, that I can see, is to claim it as a lift, and I think this is mostly a misunderstanding on the part of the average person. They do not pay attention to the things a student of lifting weights does, and wherever they see a man hold up any object by his bodily power, they offhand call it a lift. Of course, I am not overlooking the point that some unscrupulous individuals can camouflage their feats by using trickery, but I fail to see why we have to consider them when there are so many men around who can do the right thing properly. It is a fact that a person has to be schooled to a certain extent in anything before they really understand it, and while these nondescripts get away with some of their stuff, they certainly do not with those who have the slightest knowledge of what constitutes a feat of strength. Some sensational writer, every once in a while, burst into print and tries to disprove lifting in general from the feats of these men, but they only show their own lack of knowledge of the real feats which are performed and the real strength which is built by lifting and lifters.

I happened to read a book not long ago on feats of strength, and really I had to laugh. In his efforts to prove the difference between feats that are genuine, and those that are not, the author actually disclaimed genuine feats and his gullibility was proven by statements he had swallowed from others who had helped to educate him to their own advantage. Recalling one feat, the author states that one man who never weighed more than the one hundred forty pound limit, made a back lift of over six thousand pounds. I happen to know all the men personally he writes of, and I know what they can do. In the first place, the great back lifter failed at a little over nineteen hundred pounds when he was asked to prove his claim. He never did better either. My friend, Warren Lincoln Travis, promptly got under the load and played with it. The party who wrote that book was in no condition to do so, as he was not even a physical culturist, let alone a lifter, and relied upon information supplied him by others who saw their opportunity. Unintentionally, perhaps, such writers do more harm than good.

About one thousand years ago, feats of bone strength, as I will call them, were very popular at the Venetian games. Those athletes were famed for the wonderful human pyramids they built. The victory went to the team that could build the highest and hold the tableaux longest without wavering. An ancient chronicler wrote to the effect that when the order came to disband, the man on the top did a number of tricks and jumped off, each man following suit and performing their best stuff, as their turn came. What interested me mostly, was the way the chronicler finished his story. He said the bottom men, "were youths of strong bone."

We might say that bone strength is a rigid force used in resisting gravity, and muscular strength an active force resisting gravity. It is the constructional steel rigidity in a two inch steel nail driven in a piece of wood that is capable of supporting a man of one hundred eighty pounds. For their size, the bones are capable of great resistance, and as we have instances where men who performed supporting feats of strength have a limit,—as proof,—their broken limbs, and because we know the bones have great resistance, and resistance is strength, no matter in what form it is, there actually is such a thing in existence as bone strength.

CHAPTER VII
WHAT IS THE BOGEY IN FOREARM AND CALF DEVELOPMENT?

For one man that you will meet who has a fairly well built chest, you will find one hundred who have a poorly shaped pair of calves; and for every ten you find with a good looking biceps, you will find eighty with poor forearms.

The relative difference between biceps and forearm development is not so great as that which exists between the chest and calf. No doubt, this is due to the fact that when a person strives to improve the size of his upper arm, he involves to a certain extent some forearm action, which helps to bring about a little better condition. But still, the average is tremendously below what it should be, for reasons that we will go into further on in our story. Perhaps you will think it an odd comparison to try to strike an average between chest and calf development, but it is not such a bad contrast after all, if you are willing to consider the fact that the craze for chest development is almost equal to the big biceps craze, and that the legs are used continually all day long in the transportation of our body. If the chest had any kind of muscular co-ordination with the calves as the biceps has with the forearm, then we would see better results. Yet, if we had to seek a comparison of other muscles of the body with the calf and forearm, we would reach a worse average. It is the truth that no two parts of the body are concentrated upon so keenly as the chest and biceps, and no two parts are neglected so badly as the calf and forearms. It is natural for all of us to go after an object that provides the possibility of gaining the richest success, no matter what our object may be in either business or in sport. So it is just one of our worldly failings to make the same choice when it comes to muscle building.

A big chest and a big biceps are two of the greatest glories of a young man's dreams, while the forearm and calves are forgotten. There is always an awakening, which usually is brought about when the contrast between the fine development of other muscles, in comparison with the lack of development in these two quarters becomes evident. Still, developing in either of these two parts is not such an easy matter. A very few do make unusual progress. Once in a great while, I hear from some exercise fan who tells me that he has no trouble with his calves or his forearms. He usually has troubles that lie elsewhere. I generally find that nature has been very kind to these parties in the first place, but these cases are rare.

Of the two, there is no question but what the muscles of the calf are the more difficult to improve. It really is a shame that this is so. Poor calves spoil the whole build, no matter how good we may be. Somehow I have acquired the habit of always looking at the calves the first, when surveying a physique. The calf of the leg does not have to be extremely large to set off a build; it is the shapeliness that gives distinction to their appearance that counts. Well formed calves are something beautiful to look upon, and the finest examples of calf development, apart from a certain class of body builders who did not overlook the existence of these muscles in the first place, are found to belong to sprinters and cyclists. They both also have fine thighs, but their calves are generally par excellence, and this is particularly true of the bike racer. Of course, these conditions are perfectly natural, because these men depend more largely upon their leg strength for success, than do other athletes. Yet, I am not going to advise everybody who wants good calves to take up sprint racing or bike riding. There are other means just as effective, but these two examples are good to bear in mind during our lesson on muscular operation.

I have listened to various arguments, by learned individuals who each had different ideas as to where they thought the difficulty existed in these troubled sectors. Each man had a certain amount of truth behind his convictions, but I believe that it is a collection of many reasons that make the calf and forearm muscles very stubborn from a development standpoint rather than just one reason. For the present, we will consider the calf, since I appear to have first allowed my mind to run in that direction.

In the chapter in which I have discussed the mystery of strength, I have shown how nature from her natural reservoirs supplies the body with the strength to suit the needs of circumstance and how she accumulates muscular size in proportion to the stimulated strength, but here is a place where, at first appearance, nature appears to have fallen down. Take postmen or policemen, men with an occupation that calls for constant use of the legs with very little interruption for rest during the day, you rarely see any of these men with unusual muscular size, unless they have practiced some sports that have involved great calf action. Now I agree that this does not seem right, for we have found that if a man goes into the lumber camps and swings an axe, he received bigger and better shoulders, and so on, but here we find nothing out of the ordinary. The only change we can find is that the calf muscles are very hard, and they have a clearer muscular separation. There must be a reason for this peculiarity, which apparently has been overlooked, but I think that we can find it. In the first place, ordinarily, the lower legs do not have so much to do with carrying the body- weight as does the thighs. Most people have the impression that the lower limbs do it all. If they did, then nature would have equipped us with larger lower leg muscles. What actually takes place is that the muscles of the calf control the stride, the leg action from the knee down, in extending the foot. The calf muscles appear to me to be especially endowed with endurance, and they are primarily built for that purpose. In ordinary use they are called upon more for endurance than great muscular contraction. It surely is strange then that their structure should be so much harder than any of the other muscles, that is, if we view the situation in the same manner as the men who believe that hard muscles are a sure sign of being muscle bound. This one fact disproves that hard muscles are bound. It is the quality of their structure that has increased their fibrous texture, and the size they ordinarily acquire is sufficient for ordinary conditions. Under examination, it is found that the tissues of the calf muscles are considerably more dense than the muscles of the biceps

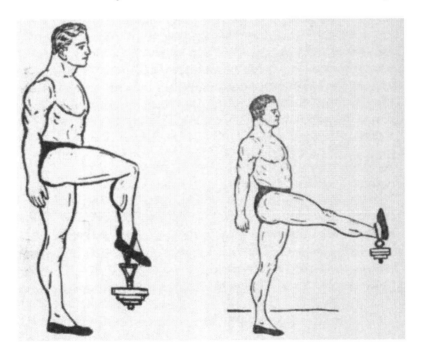

or even again, the manner in which we walk has a lot to do with it. A very well known track coach and famous walking champion, once told me that the longer the stride the less the actual action of the gastrocnemius muscle, which is the double headed muscle that forms the back of the calf, is called into play. He claimed that the greatest share of the lower leg action was absorbed by the great Achilles tendon, and the muscle that runs up the front of the shin bone. This was the reason he advanced, why walkers and long distance runners, in general, do not have larger calf muscles than they have. In the heel and toe stride, the body weight is "rocked," as walkers term it, and the real movement takes place from the hips and not from the knees. In sprint racing it is different; the action comes from the knee, as we will see. Anyone can observe that people with flat feet have poor calves, and a man with a small foot is apt to have a better shaped calf, because his stride is shorter, and he is better balanced upon his toes. This is one reason why women as a rule have better shaped calves than men. It was not so twenty years ago, because they had not then adopted, for general use, the high heeled shoes now worn. High heels cause a greater contraction of the calf muscle and also shorten the stride. Wearing such footwear is not a procedure of which I can say, I greatly approve, but it has an effect upon the calf that bolsters my belief.

People who live in the mountains have better calves than the lowlanders. Walking up a steep grade, or climbing crevices, as mountaineers do, compel a shortened stride with a greater contraction of the gastrocnemius muscles.

Nothing but very vigorous play of these muscles will increase their growth, and it has to be vigorous.

The muscles of the leg and foot are divided into three series, and are termed as follows: First series, the extensor muscles on the front of the leg and dorsum of the foot. Second series, the muscles on the lateral, or side of the leg. Third series, the flexor muscles on the back of the leg and the sole of the foot.

I am not going to name all these muscles, as most of the names do not have any special meaning, as do some others in the body. These Latin and Greek names are not the easiest thing in the world to remember, so we will just concentrate on the more important names. The gastrocnemius or "calf muscle" as I explained, lies on the back of the calf, and they are muscles of flexion, which does not exactly mean of contraction. To flex is to bend, as when we say a piece of material is very flexible, meaning bendable. They bend the lower leg on the thigh, operating much as the forearm does on the upper arm. The gastrocnemius have very powerful knee control, and are divided in two sections. Each head has an origin at the knee, but becomes inserted into a broad membranous tendon which we generally term the tendon of Achilles, although it has another name. If a person walks flat- foot, very little contraction of the muscles is caused, as it is the muscle that contracts as the body is raised high upon the toes. The next important muscle is the Peronaeus Tertius, which is really a part of the extensor digitorum longus. It is a long strip of muscle that runs down the outside of the leg. It helps to flex the ankle, and raise the foot in a lateral manner as in dancing and skating. Another muscle on the lateral part of the leg is the Peronaeus Longus, which exerts the foot and greatly strengthens the arch of the foot by its passage across the sole to its insertion.

Try to keep this clearly in mind as I am explaining the principle motions of these muscles all together, instead of separately, so we will have no interruption in studying the best type of exercises later on. The next is the Soleus, which does not cover the sole of the foot. It is a muscle that operates individually and is a very powerful extensor of the ankle with a triple origin. Our last muscle of importance is the Tibialis Anterior, better known to us as the shin bone muscle. Now these are all with which I am going to deal, because what these muscles do, actually controls and decides what the other muscles, that surround the calf, will do. We all realize that the largest muscle is that twin creation on the back of the calf, and it is the muscle that decides for us on sight, whether a person has a good looking leg or not. However, we positively must consider all the muscles when it comes to the right kind of exercise to promote growth. If you want to find out how little a person knows about calf development, ask them to give you the best exercises for the lower limb, and it is a cinch that they will know a greater variety for any other part of the body than for the calf. It is surprising to me how little is really known about exercise of the lower limbs.

To invite a person to go out and walk six miles, jump, sprint or bike race, in order to get a better leg, is to ask them to indulge in sports for which everybody has not the time or the inclination. To me, such advice seems poor indeed, or an admission that you are stumped. The real value of exercise lies in its ability to supply the need at a saving of time. Most people are not interested in the idea of taking up dancing, or sprinting to gain good legs. I know the vast majority of body builders are not. There is a lot of difference between games and exercise. Exercise is a thing which every-one can benefit from and excel at, but this is not true of games.

When I was striving for better calves, I had the same problem to face as my calves were poor for the rest of my body, and all anyone could tell me, even the most learned instructors of that time, was to raise upon the toes of both feet, then upon the toes of one foot, while holding some heavy object in my hands. I did that for years it seemed, but got nowhere, simply because the muscles became accustomed to those movements, just as they do to walking, until the movements finally resolved themselves into an endurance exercise. I began to study the muscles and how they functioned, and then I found the answer that brought my fourteen inch calves up to sixteen and a half inches. I found out long before that muscles grew better under the stimulus of a greater variety of exercises, rather than under the monotony of one or two. I arranged my program and followed the principle explained in the chapter on "How specialization destroys the jinx in stubborn muscles." One week I would do one group of calf exercises, the next week another group, and then mix them up. In other words, I exercised the calves from every conceivable angle. I would place a heavy bar bell on the back of my neck, and raise high on the toes of both feet. Then I walked around the room balanced on the toes, keeping the knees locked all the time. While holding a kettle bell in one hand, I performed the one foot raise, keeping the other foot off the floor. But I had to rest the tips of my fingers on the back of a chair, in order to preserve my balance. However, this is what I had always been doing, and my calf muscles were used to that action. I was stumped. Nobody had anything else to offer me, and much as I realized the value of games, I had not the time at my disposal to practice them. Then again, it was winter and the roads were blocked with snow. I obtained a book on anatomy, and read underneath the explanatory construction of the gastrocnemius, the short line "Flexor of the knee and extensor of the ankle." Not much on which to work, but somehow I puzzled over the way the word "flexor" was used. Even now, the majority of exercise teachers still have the misguided habit of using flexion and contractions of muscles as though they had the same meaning, which is all wrong. The difference began to dawn on me, and I then understood that a flexion is a bending process, not a contraction, although it involves such muscular effort. You can tense and flex your ankle, wrist and other joints, but you can't contract them. Everything came to me with a rush. I understood better why walkers and distance runners, had not the calf development of sprinters and bike riders. The flexion of the knee is much more powerful in the latter than in the former, although the sprinter and bike rider use the muscles a trifle differently. A sprinter races on the ball of his foot with his weight carried forward, and as he makes his leg drives, he brings his knee almost up to the chest, thereby bringing into action more forcibly the gastrocnemius muscles. He is actually striving to see how fast he can leap ahead with his weight. A bike rider goes through even more powerful leg movements. He straps his feet to the pedals, so that he is better able to "pull" the big driving wheel around, as well as thrust it forwards and drive it downwards. It is claimed that the "pull" round is what gives them their terrific speed, hence the remarkable calf display.

I lined up a few new exercises with this knowledge in mind hoping that they would give me the same results without being obliged to indulge in those sports. In place of a dancing school, I adopted the footwork of Kid McCoy, "The Dancing Master" making the play a little more

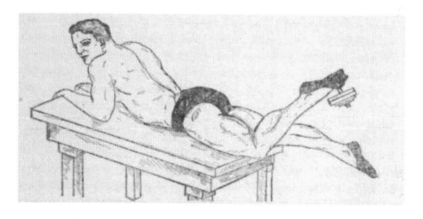

vigorous by using a dumb-bell in each hand. I believe I have explained this practice before in the columns of "Strength." However, there is no harm in telling it again. I arranged a circle, marked off in squares, each square being numbered. I took up my position in the center, balanced upon the toes in a squat position. That is, I was almost sitting on my heels. You can spring faster that way. A friend would call out any number he saw fit, and I would leap to it; from one to the other, backwards, forwards, and sideways, always on the rebound. It was great stuff for the eye, mind and wind as well as muscle. Then I would walk up and down a flight of stairs once, while holding a kettle bell in each hand. The only trouble with this last exercise is that it tires you out too quickly, because there is so much thigh action. But a little of it is good. Now here is something which I learned. The fact that you raise high on one foot with the knee locked is not proof that you bring about a complete contraction of the gastrocnemius. Nearly every muscle culturist believes this is the case, but it is not so. It gives great play to the lateral muscles, and will make the calf look deep when viewed sideways, but will not give the width, which is the appearance so desirable to the leg culturist. The outer part of the gastrocnemius secures a greater amount of play than the inner part, and you must remember, this muscle is a powerful flexor of the knee and extensor of the ankle, which means, in order to give the gastrocnemius its fullest contraction, the knee must be bent, and the ankle extended. Try this one. Tie a dumb-bell of about fifteen to twenty-five pounds with a cloth around the ankle, then place the hands on the hips. Gradually draw the knee up to the chest, and as you do so point the toe to the floor. This will give complete contraction to both parts of the twin muscle, besides giving the desired effect upon the inner head to promote width as well as depth. Here is another that will get the inner head by just an ankle extension. Hitch a light kettle bell of about ten pounds to the toes, place one hand on the back of a chair, just to safeguard the balance of the body, then begin by raising the leg forward, keeping the toe pointed as much as possible.

Going back to the position, as given in the last exercise, but one, with the knee raised high, from that position allow the toes to travel in a straight line inwards and outwards. A few movements like this will make you feel happily contented that you are on the right road at last.

A real good exercise is in something like an exercise I give for the development of the biceps of the thighs. Lie face downwards on a table, and allow a friend to place a kettle bell over each foot. Extend the ankle by bending the heel backwards and pointing the toes. Begin to curl the foot towards the buttock. As the foot is lowered, still keep the toes pointed. Practice this exercise with both feet working together, and then each foot alternately.

To develop the muscle on the shin bone, stand erect and hitch the foot into a kettle bell handle, then raise the leg to right angles with the body, but this time don't point the toe. Instead, bend the foot towards the shin bone. Deep knee bending with the feet flat on the floor is also a good exercise for the shin muscles. I might add, that this muscle is one that walkers do have very well developed.

Did you ever try raising on the ball of the foot and every few counts change the angle of the feet, so that one time they will be pointed out, and then work so the toes are turned in considerably?

There is still another exercise that puts pep and muscle in the calf, which I should mention, although it takes quite a bit of practice to be able to perform it correctly. It is the Russian ballet step, where you squat upon the haunches with arms folded and balance on the ball of the foot. Hop backwards, sideways and forwards, and when you get accustomed to the step, walk forward, and as each step is taken, straighten out one leg. It is rather difficult, but if you are interested in securing a better calf appearance, you will find it well worth your time and patience.

I dwelt longer on this subject than I intended, but I feel sure you will profit by it. I have had many pupils tell me that these exercises have done for them in a few weeks what years of practice failed to yield. One pupil of mine, actually increased his calf measurement from twelve and three-quarter inches to fifteen and a half inches, inside of two months. When I think of how I slaved for mine, I envy the young exercise fan who can start right off and know he is on the right road for results. However, I am glad to know that my experiences have been able to help others succeed. That alone is worth a lot to me. One thing I must impress upon your mind, and that is the value of massage in the building of the calf muscles. After every exercise period, massage them thoroughly. Always keep them as loose and as pliable as possible.

The forearm bogey is a pig with another snout, as we used to say. Where the calves become hard from constant use, the forearm muscles do not. With the exception of the mechanic, the average person seldom stirs up much forearm action. In the first place he objects to carrying anything that is heavy, and in the second place anything carried is generally with a bent arm, so that any physical effort is taken care of by the upper arm muscles. The forearms are usually soft and flabby, and it takes a little while before this enervated tissue can reconstruct itself.

However, among mechanics we find very much the same condition of forearms as we find to be true of the legs of the policeman or postman. They do the same thing all the time, use their muscles in the one routine. The muscles grow sufficiently strong for their work, and there it all ends. Of course, in extremely laborious occupations, such as using a pick and shovel, trundling a loaded wheelbarrow or handling bales, etc., in a shipping house, we find many fine examples of forearm development. But it was the old time blacksmith of Longfellow's day, when forgings were heavy and more often used, and made with no other mechanical help than the heavy hammer and the brawn of the arm, that gave us the finest pattern of the mighty arm. But those days are gone, and anyhow none of us want to slave at such laborious occupations in order to possess a fine pair of arms. Exercise we will do and with pleasure, say all the muscle seekers. Just show us the way. This I can easily do and in a manner that will give you lots of fun, while you are striving for profit.

Forearm development was easy for me. It seemed I always had it, and I had to do the reverse of the majority, make my biceps grow in proportion to my forearm. But I attribute all my forearm development to the pleasant exercises I practiced, that always kept me playing, as it were.

Like everybody else, I admire a fine arm, and I would like to see every body culturist with a pair. Legs like John Lemm, Joe Urlacher, Moss, Manger, and Passannant, and arms like Saxon, Nordquest, Aston and Cadine. That's what I like to see. Shape, size, and strength.

There is no bogey in calf or forearm development; it is just certain conditions that have to be overcome, and this can be done with proper exercise. In my next chapter I am going to discuss at length how you really can beautify your body with a real pair of arms, equal to the calves I know you are going to have after you have practiced the exercises in this lesson a short while. Use whatever weight dumb-bells, bar bells and kettle bells you feel comfortably able to handle. Always let your physical condition be your guide in exercise and you will succeed.

CHAPTER VIII
THICKENING THE WRIST BY
STRENGTHENING THE GRIP

You will notice in the previous chapter, that although I set out to find the bogey in forearm and calf development, I did not write much about the forearms. Towards the close of the chapter, I did call your attention to them, but I purposely let the subject slide for different reasons, all of which revolve around the fact that so little seems to be known about successful calf and forearm building. It must be this, otherwise we would not be so everlastingly confronted with complaints of failure from so many who crave muscle upon these two sectors. If there is a bogey, it is in lack of knowledge, and in absolutely nothing else. I devoted practically the whole of the last chapter to calf construction, and I find if I am to give you the best forearm information, it is going to take at least two chapters. But I believe your interest is strong enough to stand it, as I know you will find much refreshing information as your interest will be centered around new material.

The title of this chapter may lead you to believe that the forearm is not going to be very much discussed in this chapter after all; but it is, and thoroughly. I chose that title because I want you to get the idea out of your head, that you have to own large wrists before you can own a better and larger forearm. It is the forearm that makes the wrist, rather than the wrist making the forearm. I have listened to the wails of scores of young men who lament that they will never have a decent forearm because their wrist is far too small; and that is the accepted idea. But it is wrong. You have to get the forearm first, and in order to get the forearm you have to get the grip. We always see a powerful clasp go hand in glove with a strong forearm. However, you can readily recall many friends who apparently have a strong hand clasp but no unusual forearm size. That is true. You will find salesmen have a hand clasp above the average, but they specialize on that grip only, and are often on the lookout to take a quick grip and secure an advantage over the ordinary person, who usually is not interested in hand clasping resistance. Yet there is no denying the fact that when these worthies shake hands, the wrist ligaments are fairly prominent. On the other hand, they soon know when they meet a strong armed man. There is something in a strong clasp.

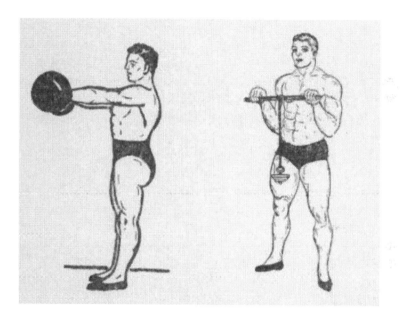

Everything we pick up in our hands calls for a certain amount of grip. That grip calls into motion the forearm muscles, and the ligaments of these muscles control the wrist and hand movements. This is the case and the common assumption that the wrist controls the forearm and the grip of the hand is all wrong. Your grip will always be measured by the amount of forearm strength you have, and your ability to carry objects and raise them off the floor. So in order to increase the forearm muscles, we have to cultivate our gripping qualities to their fullest, and the wrist will be taken care of automatically.

It has taken up a large number of words to tell you what I mean when I say "get away from the idea because your wrist only measures six and a half inches or seven inches, that it has placed a fatal seal on your possibilities for forearm growth." Get over this idea that a very ordinary fellow you know having naturally a seven and three-quarter inch wrist has it all over you. This is not so. I don't say you will make an eight inch wrist out of six inch wrist, but I know you can improve it a lot, and its quality will manifest itself in the strength and shapeliness of your forearms. Many people naturally have very heavy bones around the wrist. Well, you can't offset that, but you can acquire thicker wrist cables, and the bones will slightly increase their structure, from resistance, as it is applied in its proper place.

A lot of exercisers write to me to complain that when they do that certain leg exercise where they straddle a bar bell and hold it in the hands while they do a slight knee bend, their grip plays out before their legs get their workout. In their mind, it is always their poor grip, but they are mistaken; as the forearm strength and hand grip of no man was ever sufficient to cope with the vigorous play of which the large hip and thigh muscles are capable. There is too much disparity in the relative strength of these separate members of the body. The best way to overcome this, so that the legs get the best results, is to make a harness of canvas to fit over the head and rest upon the shoulders, with a hook sewn in at each end. You simply allow the bar bell to lie in the hooks, and the body supports the weight instead of the grip. Some have more trouble, than they ordinarily should, with this exercise. They find that the weight straightens their fingers out and pulls away. This cause is as much the lack of finger strength as of the hand grip, but the

100

next chapter is going to be devoted to the cultivation of finger strength, so I will stick to my initial discussion.

There are numerous muscles in the forearm, which are classified as pronators, extensor and flexor muscles. The pronators are the muscles of rotation, while the extensors straighten out the arm, and the flexor bends the forearm upon the upper arm. Taking our first survey on the anterior forearm, which is the front, we find four muscles that have a common origin, on the extreme end of the humerus bone, at the elbow joint. They divide and spread, to compose the bulk of muscle so pronounced on a well developed arm. It is the second muscle from the inside that has the largest bulk of the four, and possesses the roundness which gives the canoe like shape to the front of the forearm when in repose, and is more forcibly evident when flexed. They are some of the pronator muscles and flexors. The muscles on the dorsal part of the arm are seven in number, and included among these is the supinator longus, also known as the Brachio-Radialis, which is the most important extensor muscle in the forearm. Running by its side is the Extensor Carpi Radialis Longus, which is the accessory extensor muscle that co-operates with the supinator.

The great peculiarity of our forearm muscles is the strange way in which they are capable of twisting. The supinator longus and its accessory muscle have a remarkable spiral twist to them. It arises from the humerus bone (on which the biceps rests) underneath the bicep, but twists over the outside of the elbow joint to become attached to the front of the forearm. I am inclined to believe that the supinator longus is the most important muscle in the forearm. It is capable of rotating, flexing, and powerful in extending or straightening the arm. It sets an arm off also, giving breadth to the arm at the elbow when viewed sideways. Did you ever notice the arm of a pick and shovel laborer or a man who is accustomed to carry objects in his hands? For instance, a railroad porter. Of course the majority of porters keep their arms covered, with his arms bared carrying a heavy object but if you ever see one, just notice the forearm at the elbow and you will see what appears like a deep indentation and then a hump of muscle. That is the effect this muscle gives to the arm when an object is being carried. On the arms of porters, it often is pronounced, and also upon laborers. Just

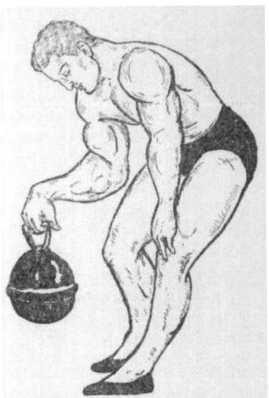

clench your fists, and thrust your arms straight down by the sides, then bend the wrist back to the outside, and notice how this muscle stands out. Yet another interesting way to view this muscle is to bend the arm so that the fist rests upon the chest. Bend the arm more forcibly upon the biceps by employing the other hand, and the muscle will accentuate greatly. Then while in this position, twist the wrist and just notice how firmly it becomes tensed in the process of a wrist rotary movement. When a weight is raised overhead, and held at full arms' length, it is this muscle and its accessory muscle that do all the work, co-operating with the triceps of the upper arm. The other muscles being flexors should never be employed to any extent when raising a weight overhead, as they counteract the extensors.

The muscles on the front of the arm, being flexors, apply their force more powerfully in movements that bend the arm at the elbow. Their contraction is even greater whenever any object is being raised towards the shoulder while the hand is bent at the wrist, downwards. Forearm builders liken this position of the arm to a swan's neck, as it is the position which a youngster will form with his arm when patterning a swan on a shadow screen. This is why, when advising a person to practice a movement with the wrist turned downwards, the movement is termed a swan's neck formation.

It is the flexor muscles on the front of the arm and the supinator muscles that are always the least developed among beginners. It is in these regions that muscle builders, with poor arms, fall down. Well, we cannot blame them too much, because like calf exercises, they only seem to know one or two exercises, and that ends it. When a person becomes more familiar with the uses of these muscles, he can see that something else, in the way of exercise, has to be done. I am satisfied that if any of you follow out the advice I am going to give, you will soon be piling up muscle on those stick pin arms.

You may wonder how your wrist will become improved by any forearm practice, so before we go any further let me enlighten you upon the fact that the muscles all taper off into ligaments. The weaker the muscles, the more stringy and thin are these cables. The stronger and bulkier they build up, the thicker the ligaments become. As these ropes of connection taper off at the. wrist, it is only a natural condition that the wrist size should be increased.

When I commenced heavy exercise, I only had a seven inch wrist, just an average size as I have said, but to-day my wrist measures every bit of eight and a half inches. The sinews that have massed upon the wrist are very heavy, and have powerful contraction, and perhaps I am justified in the joy I take in my forearm strength, shape, and size. It measures fifteen and a quarter inches. I practiced many forms of exercise to which I owe my success in arm molding. In one of my writings I have made the statement that forearm growth never seemed hard for me to secure. The truth of the fact is this, although I certainly did a lot of work on my forearms, yet I never actually noticed it. You see the exercises I performed were more in the line of stunts, and I played at them as you would a game. These stunts were a never failing source of interest and pleasure to me, that reminds me of the old saw that we never do anything so well as the things we like. Unfortunately, exercise has a tendency to become monotonous, especially when the number of exercises are limited, and as I have inferred before, I believe that reason is the cause for lack of calf and forearm development—lack of knowledge. Exercise must never be a grind; it must be a pleasure, and have the qualifying results to always supply the urge.

When I was a young boy, we did not have the variety of fine outfits the present day body culturist finds. We used to play a lot with block weights of different weights. The half hundred weight was the most popular, and I well remember that my first strongman outfit consisted of a very short piece of a broken steel shaft, that weighed about forty pounds and was about three inches in diameter. A very unwieldy implement for a fifteen year old boy, you will admit. My other "weapon" was an old half hundred pound block weight. With these implements I commenced my adventures into strengthland with visions of myself as Hercules not far ahead. As time went on, I became very adept in handling this block weight, and when I was sixteen years of age I could duplicate all of the regular feats with ease. Of course, most of these stunts involve a good grip, but while I did not have this valuable asset in the first place, I gradually acquired it from training. The shape and size of the hands have a lot to do with many of these feats. Some people naturally have large hands, which give them a greater gripping space, but my hands were only of the average size. The hand itself is broad, but the fingers are short. It was not much of a handicap, and I figured that we cannot have everything; so it is up to each of us to make the best of what we have, and offer no excuses.

The regular grip and forearm exercise really was a bore to me. I could not see the idea of holding the arms straight out in front, winding up a weight tied on a stick. My shoulders always became tired before I got the right effect upon the forearm, so I changed it a little, on the principle that the muscles intended for that exercise should be the flexors of the front forearm; yet by holding both arms straight out in front, the action was being absorbed just as much, if not more, by the supinator extensors. Just as the gastrocnemius of the calf have greater contraction when the knee is flexed, I figured the same thing would happen to the forearm. Instead of holding the arms straight out, I bent them considerably at the elbow, until the formation of the arm with the body represented the letter V. I found I could handle much more weight this way, which gave a more powerful play to the flexor muscles, and all the former shoulder fatigue was eliminated. Where before I found thirty pounds tired my shoulders and not my forearms, I could then handle fifty pounds with the right effort directed upon the proper quarters.

Most exercise fans imagine that chinning the bar with both hands is entirely a biceps developer. It certainly has a splendid effect upon the upper arm, but it also gives the forearm very vigorous play. This was also part of my practice, with the following variations. Suppose I was going to chin myself a dozen times. I would divide the repetitions in this manner. Catching the bar with both hands in the regular grip, I would chin three times, then reverse one hand, so that one palm was facing me and the other would be turned away. Next three chins would see both hands reversed, so that both palms were facing me. The last three chins I would do entirely differently; taking hold of the bar with the regular grip, but with the forearms crossed, in a position so that the right hand would be where the left grip would be ordinarily taken, and the left hand would be in the regular right hand place. This chin is rather difficult and calls for a lot of arm strength. In the first place, your hands cannot be spaced much apart, and you will not be able to chin your weight so high. At the same time you will find that your body has a tendency to spin around. The fact that you have to fight these conditions is just what will bring the most out in your arm development. It is not necessary to practice these chins in the rotation I have just given. I would do the hardest first, and leave the easiest for the last, which will be hard enough as you tire. My main object was to see how well I could chin instead of how many times. Too many young chaps figure it is greater to chin thirty times than fifteen. Numerically it is, but the results are not the same. The chinning fiend chins fast, and swings his body to aid the pulls, but that is no good. Too much lost motion. I would rather have twenty-five correct chins as my record, than fifty otherwise. When a bunch of enthusiasts would get together, we would tie weights on the feet and see who could chin with the most weight. A heavy man will not chin as many times, or handle as much weight on his feet, but we always made a weight allowance in such a case. I remember some of the boys could chin with a friend hanging around their waist. Anyhow these stunts certainly improve the grip and the forearm. Just try them for yourself.

Many enthusiasts claim that their wrists are too flexible to allow them to perform many ordinary movements of the forearms. Now I hope this statement will not convey to you the idea that a wrist should be almost rigid in order to be strong. A strong wrist is always flexible. The difference is that the weak wrist has no control over its flexibility, which invites wrist strain, when the wrist is bent beyond a certain angle. The strong arm man always has control. Just notice the acute angle to which the weight lifters and hand balancers are capable of bending their wrists, and yet have them under wonderful control. It is all in the strength of your forearm muscles and their ligaments. The novice in hand balancing always feels a stiffness at the wrist when making his first few hand stands on the floor, but practice accustoms the wrist to bend to the angle and strengthens it. The same applies in heavy weight lifting, which is the reason why bar bell users have powerful wrists.

It annoys me to see a novice wear wrist straps. It is so unnecessary and unnatural. Your muscles were made for A purpose and that was not to wear wrist straps. They only tend to weaken the wrist by absorbing the resistance that the ligaments require, which keep the wrist weak and prone to strain. If you have strained the wrist, that is different, but cold water bandages will relieve the strain and help toughen the sinews. Don't use a wrist strap any longer than necessary. Professional athletes only wear them for show purposes, to set off the looks of their arm, and the material is always of light flexible leather. Strengthen your wrist by natural means.

In passing, I might mention that it is the downward pressure upon the bones of the arms, as involved in lifting heavy weights and hand balancing, that increases the thickness of the bone structure.

Here is a clever exercise for the grip and wrist, which makes the pronator muscles of the forearm go the limit and also develops a spectacular stunt. Grasp a bar of about fifteen or twenty pounds in the center by the right hand; give the bar a twist to the left, and allow it to make a full circle before you catch it with the left hand. Immediately the left hand grasps it, let it go from your right hand, as the

107

right hand will have travelled the limit of its rotary extent. You simply catch the bar with the left hand long enough for the right hand to untwist and catch it in its natural hold. It looks as though both hands are operating, but it really is the right arm that is doing it all. The left hand is just an accessory. Always catch with the left hand above the right hand, and be sure to allow the bar to make a full circle before you change hands. It looks great when you get it down so pat that the spins are rapid enough to make the "whirlwind circle" as the feat is named. Do not practice with one arm only. Give both arms their share, and you will find a great kick is supplied to the pronator muscles.

A variation of this is practiced by using only one hand. However, in this it is necessary to support the elbow on the hip. As the wrist reaches the limit of its turn, give the bar a slight heave and catch it as it circles. When you get good at this, you can use both hands. As one circle is made and the grip of the right hand is released, the left hand catches and gives a turn, keeping the bar going from one hand to another. Before you practice any of these more advanced feats, train yourself by holding a light bar in the hand and allowing the bar to revolve, twisting the wrist as far as possible; then stop the twist without letting go, and turn the bar back again. Do it slowly. It is just a series of to and fro circles made by the wrist. Keep the elbow on the hip as a support and an aid throughout the practice.

In a minor way, twisting a dumb-bell has the same effect upon the pronators. For the supinator longus and its accessory muscle, a splendid exercise is performed by standing erect with the feet together, and a bar bell of twenty-five pounds, hanging at arms' length, held in front, across the thighs. From this position you slowly raise the bar bell in a quarter circle until the arms lie parallel with the shoulders.

As the bell is raised, bend the hands upwards upon the wrist. The reverse of the swan neck formation. It is the position of the hands that controls your success. Keep perfectly straight, and do not bend backwards or seek to aid the raising of the bar bell with any swing from the body. The arms must be locked at the elbow so that they are straight, and another little thought to remember is that the movement is just as effective when lowering the bell as when raising it. Although the main purpose of the exercise is to develop the supinator longus, yet it is a fine exercise for the whole body.

For the muscles on the outside, or dorsal side of the arm, the following exercise will be found effective. Stand erect while holding a dumb-bell in each hand averaging anywhere from fifteen to twenty-five pounds each, according to your strength. Let the arms hang by your sides and before you begin the exercise bend the hand upon the wrist backwards. Then begin to raise the arms up sideways. It is not necessary that they should be raised so high that they reach the level of the shoulders. Raise them as high as you can, as it is the forearm muscular action you want. When you get beyond half way to the level of the shoulders, the triceps and deltoids begin to take the aggressive, and you should not be interested in deltoid and triceps development when practicing this exercise. You can tell if you are doing it correctly, as the ends of the dumb- bells should lie horizontal with each other throughout, not endways to the floor. But the important part is how the hand is bent. You cannot watch that point too closely. If the hand is held too straight with the forearm, you will feel a wrist strain; if it is in the correct position you will feel a strong muscular contraction.

One time a friend of mine was showing me through a foundry where he was employed, and on our tour of inspection he remarked, knowing I was interested in well formed muscles, that he would show me a wonderful pair of arms. Coming to one part of the foundry he drew my attention to a man who was picking up various metal castings and placing them upon a low truck. He surely had fine forearms and the muscles on the front of his forearm bulged massively. There were a number of block weights all ranged on the floor, which this workman began to place on the truck. As he did so, I noticed how the flexors of the anterior forearm displayed themselves. I continued to watch him, but he never tired, and right away it flashed through my mind how he got those forearms. He was stooped over most of the time, and never raised the weights over waist level. This naturally gave the strongest play to the flexors, and from that lesson I devised the exercise of pulling the kettle bell to the chest, keeping the elbow close to the side, and bending the hand upon the wrist with a swan neck formation. I would steady myself by placing the disengaged hand upon the corresponding knee, and lift the kettle bell from between the feet as many times as I was comfortably able with a poundage of fifty pounds up; and the thicker the bar, the greater gripping strength is demanded. Men with large hands and long fingers can encircle thicker bars, although a person can use too thick a bar.

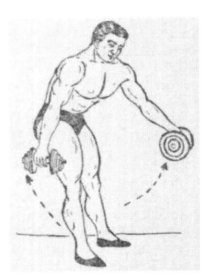

The block weight can supply many fine arm tests, which incidentally build up the arm. You know what I mean by a block weight, I suppose. It is a square piece of iron scooped out on one side with a bar inset, by which it is lifted. They weigh around fifty pounds and are generally used for testing scales. The object is to be able to grip them tight enough so that the bar does not revolve in your hand, and allow the weight to rest on the side of the arm, which is not very pleasant.

Some of the stunts you will find interesting, so I will explain a few. One of the easiest is to sit on the floor with the block weight by your side, and with a pure arm movement, raise it off the floor over the first leg. Touch the floor between the legs, then pass over the far leg and touch the floor, and return in the same manner. However, to do it right you must not allow the weight to touch the legs, and you must seek no aid from the body by swinging with the motion. Next, pull it to the shoulder and press it overhead keeping the weight all the time above the hand. A very difficult feat with which I have stuck most of the strongmen is done like this. I would stand erect with the block, or scale weight, hanging by the side, and by arm strength curl the weight with the hand bent down in swan neck fashion. After I had bent the forearm upon the upper arm as much as possible, I would pause; and with a pure wrist movement,—no shoulder action—I gripped the bar and twisted the weight so that the weight was balanced by the grip above the hand, and the hand straight with the arm. Then I would lower the weight without bending the elbow, just the wrist, and raise it back again, then describe a circle with a rotary hand movement. Another real feat is to raise the block weight from the side, keeping the wrist straight with the forearm and the weight in the same straight line, with the hand and forearm. Raising the weight until it is at right angles with the body, but the feat lies in never losing

control of the weight. An easier one is to sit on a chair and raise the block weight off the floor, and
place it on the table by your side without raising off the chair or using the other arm.

One of the greatest feats of hand grip and forearm strength I ever ran up against was in a blacksmith shop. It was an old feat practiced around the blacksmith's forge in the days when the smith was looked upon as the true personification of real strength. Many wonderful feats were seen and others talked of in the gleam of the old smithy forge, but with the decay of that picturesque occupation many of the kings of the iron arm passed.

In the old days, anvils were made in various sizes, and in a smithy shop you could always find three or four of different weights. A light anvil would be about seventy-five or eighty pounds and used for straightening nails, or light riveting. The others averaged around one hundred forty pounds to one hundred sixty-eight pounds. Where heavy forging was done, anvils much heavier were used, but the last two named seemed to be the regular thing. If any new comer wanted to try his strength they would ask him if he could lift an anvil with one hand. This was done by standing the anvil on end with the horn pointing upwards. The horn is a very thick conical affair that runs abruptly to a point. You were supposed to take hold of the horn with the hand and raise it off the floor. I have seen several raise the seventy- five or eighty pound anvil high off the floor, but I only saw two ever lift the one hundred forty pounds anvil; while on three occasions I successfully raised the anvil of one hundred and sixty-eight pounds. It is a very severe arm test, and if a man had the grip to raise any of these anvils in this manner, he always had the forearm to make it possible and the wrist to sustain the both.

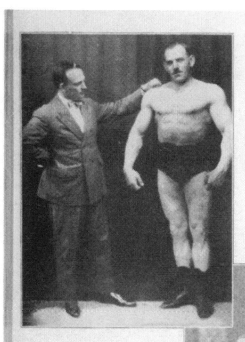

Tromp Van Diggelen, introducing Herman Gorner, the greatest man of might and muscle of all times. Greater than Cyr, Apollon, or Saxon. He has brought forward with him a new era in which the clean cut type is combined with incredible strength. Six feet one inch and 245 pounds, he has power without limit.

Louis Attila, known as the Great Attila. He is responsible for the advent of Eugene Sandow, Warren L. Travis, Lionel Strongfort and many other men of might, besides being a remarkable performer.

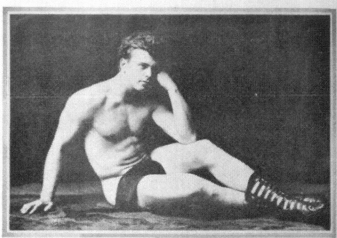

A pleasing pose by
Arthur F. Gay, of
Rochester, New York;
clever poseur and
strength athlete.

An early photo of Henry
Steinborn, in which is
forcibly evidenced the
mighty latent strength,
with which he later elec-
trified the world of
strength.

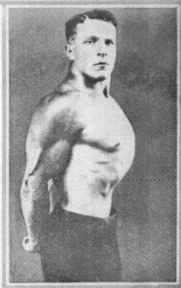

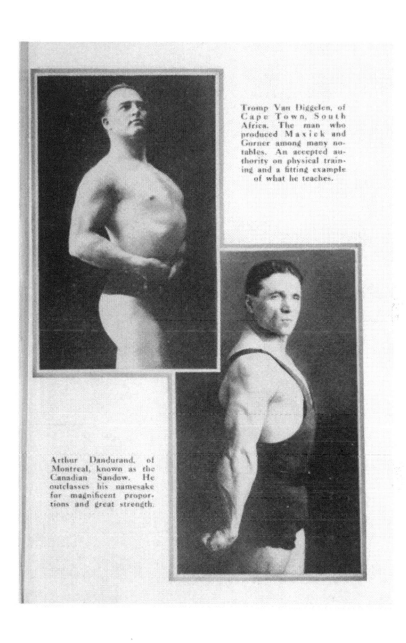

Tromp Van Diggelen, of Cape Town, South Africa. The man who produced Maxick and Gorner among many notables. An accepted authority on physical training and a fitting example of what he teaches.

Arthur Dandurand, of Montreal, known as the Canadian Sandow. He outclasses his namesake for magnificent proportions and great strength.

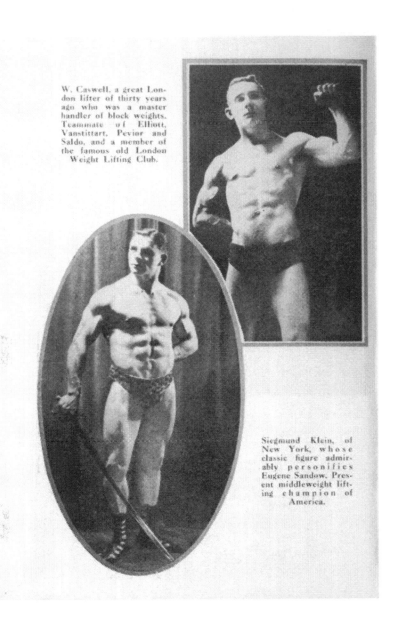

W. Caswell, a great London lifter of thirty years ago who was a master handler of block weights. Teammate of Elliott, Vanstittart, Pevior and Saldo, and a member of the famous old London Weight Lifting Club.

Siegmund Klein, of New York, whose classic figure admirably personifies Eugene Sandow. Present middleweight lifting champion of America.

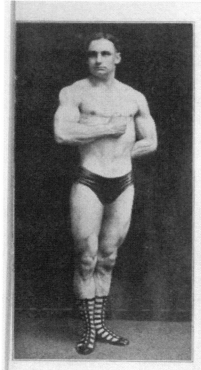

Poise, muscular balance and efficiency p a r excellence is clarified in every line of this perfectly built athlete, Charles MacMahon, o f Philadelphia; probably most prominent poseur in America, and a teacher of exceptional merit.

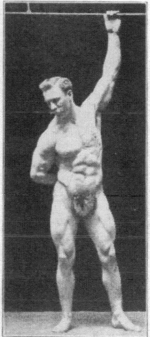

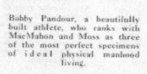

Bobby Pandour, a beautifully built athlete, who ranks with MacMahon and Moss as three of the most perfect specimens of i d e a l physical manhood living.

Katie Sandwina, a woman who descended from a long line of "strong" performers. Undoubtedly she stands out as the strongest woman in the world, combining the three qualities rarely ever seen in a strong woman. Beauty, shape and strength. It is claimed that she officially performed a Two Hands Clean and Jerk of 286 pounds. Her son inherits the characteristic of his mother, and is rated as a coming world's boxing champion.

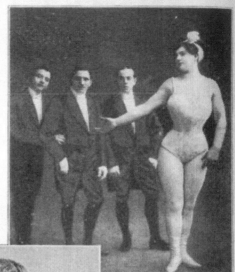

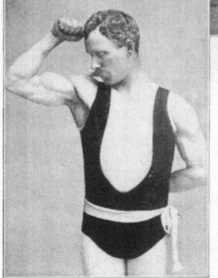

Atlas, a Welsh lightweight who claims a One Hand Clean and Jerk of 200 pounds. He is the brother of Vulcana, a woman who ranked second only to Sandwina, as a strong woman. Children of a Welsh minister, they delighted thousands with their feats a few years back.

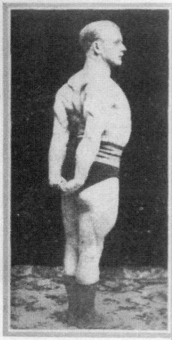

Henri Graf, a phenomenal Swiss featherweight lifter and Olympic champion.

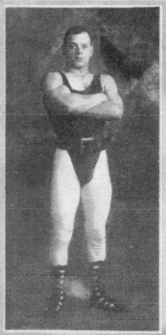

Oscar Marineau, of Montreal, a brilliant lightweight performer. At 139 pounds he lifted 266 pounds in the Two Hands Clean and Jerk. Latest reports give him credit for a Bent Press of 253 pounds. In the Two Hands Anyhow he succeeded in doing over 300 pounds.

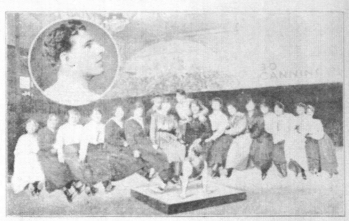

Richard Appleton a powerful 168 pound English athlete in a fine supporting feat. Appleton has done 620 pounds in the Hands Alone lift, and 220 pounds in the Two Hands Military Press.

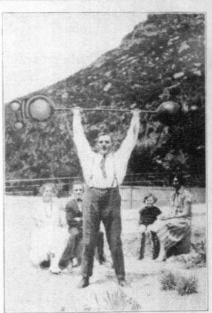

The prodigious Herman Gorner performing an impromptu Push lift with 260 pounds, while standing in loose sand.

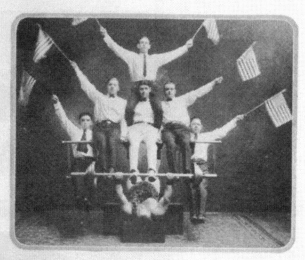

This supporting feat by Carl Moerke looks very spectacular.

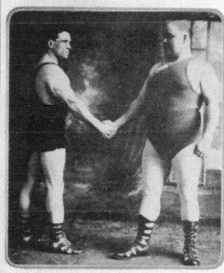

The two famous Canadian strong men, Arthur Dandurand on the left, the Canadian Sandow, and Arthur Giroux, the Montreal Hercules on the right, shaking hands prior to the opening lift in their recent contest.

Joseph Coryn, of Pittsburgh, Pennsylvania, who thirty years ago was the most colorful American strongman. Known as the American Sandow, he was idolized by Pittsburghers.

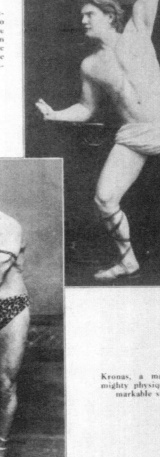

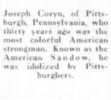

Kronas, a man with a mighty physique and remarkable strength.

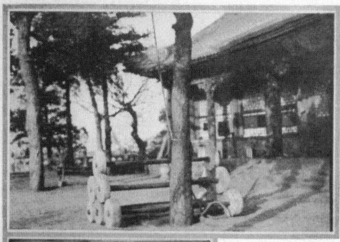

How Chinese youths
are trained. A custom
that dates back to
Confucius.

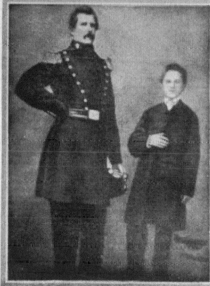

Angus McAskill, one
of the very few giants
who was known to be
terrifically strong in
proportion to his
height. He stood seven
feet nine inches and
weighed 560 pounds.
By his side is a Nova
Scotia minister, who
stood six feet three
inches.

Joseph Urlacher, of Rochester, New York, one of America's greatest light heavyweight wrestling and weight lifting stars. This picture does not do his magnificent physique justice, but he is a wonderful testimony of what bar bell training will do for a man past thirty.

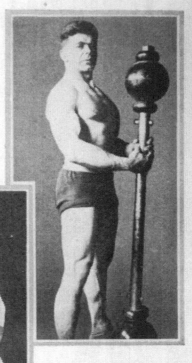

Apollon, the famous French giant, as he was at sixteen years of age. Like Elliott and Gorner, he proves that progressive bar bell training can successfully be taken up early in life. All these men are living, and at sixty-five years of age, Apollon is still a pillar of might and muscle.

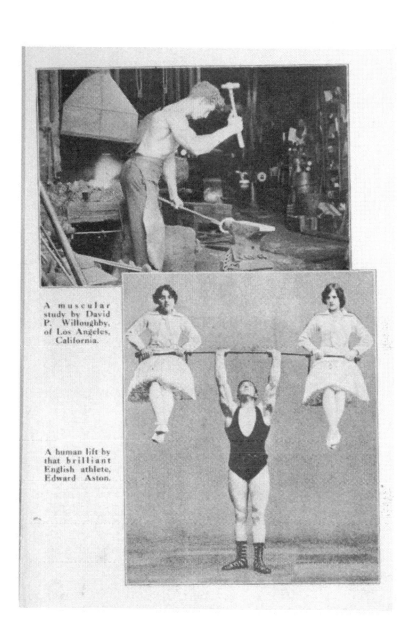

A muscular study by David P. Willoughby, of Los Angeles, California.

A human lift by that brilliant English athlete, Edward Aston.

Arthur Saxon, the "Iron Master," is revered wherever feats of strength are spoken. His two arm lift of 448 pounds and his one arm lift of 371 pounds still dazzles the world of weights.

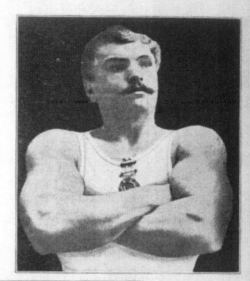

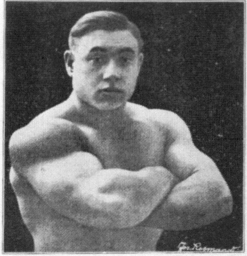

Charles Rigoulot, the young Parisian Poilu, whose marvelous ability in the Two Hands Clean and jerk and the Two Hands Snatch borders on the miraculous. Latest reports give him credit for a Two Hands Snatch of 289 pounds. He claims he will yet do 300 pounds!!!

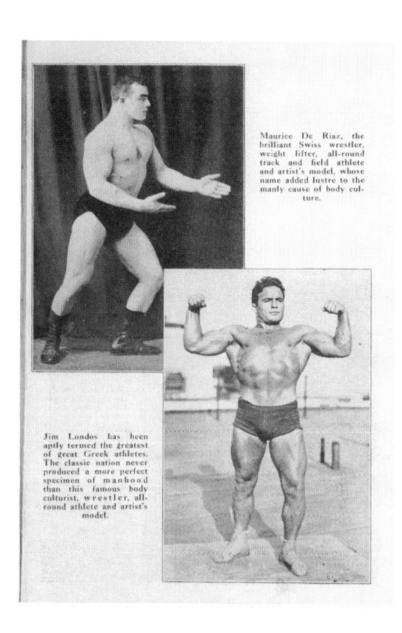

Maurice De Riaz, the brilliant Swiss wrestler, weight lifter, all-round track and field athlete and artist's model, whose name added lustre to the manly cause of body culture.

Jim Londos has been aptly termed the greatest of great Greek athletes. The classic nation never produced a more perfect specimen of manhood than this famous body culturist, wrestler, all-round athlete and artist's model.

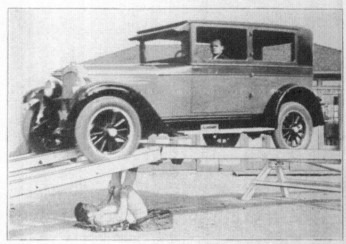

Henry Steinborn performing a mighty feat of strength at Los Angeles, California. The machine actually stopped over Henry before it ran off the platform.

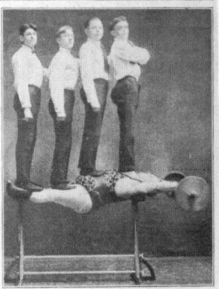

Carl Moerke, the West Haven, Connecticut German in a feat that is as unusual as it is extraordinary.

CHAPTER IX
The Value of Finger Strength and How It Is Acquired

The fingers, hand, wrist and forearm, more or less operate together, but as I told you in my last chapter, I was obliged to divide my talk on forearm development into two chapters, in order to give you the full benefits of the known facts. The only difference is that the exercises advised for developing the grip, wrist and forearm, are different from the methods employed in stimulating finger strength. Then again, because you have a strong good looking forearm, it does not necessarily mean that you really possess great finger strength; although it does mean that more often, than not. Anyhow, when I have a lot to tell you on one subject, I like to divide it so your mind is not crowded with too much information. I feel that you grasp the details better.

"Finger strength has a great deal to do with the strength of the three other subjects just discussed, and I think we will find that a little attention given to the fingers will be well worth your while.

Have you ever wondered when you were listening to a pianist interpret some difficult music, whether he had strong fingers or not? You know he has a certain amount of endurance, but perhaps that is no more than is usually found in a person who specializes on one thing. However, I have often asked myself that question, and while I knew the average pianist was not the equal of a laborer for strong fingers, I believe that the first class pianist must have more than ordinary finger strength. Of course, it would be a waste of time to look for big wrists, strong forearms and a powerful grip, as a proof of this in a pianist, as they only train their fingers, and as a rule they are not interested in strength or size, so never train with that object in view. I once happened to be talking with a man who is a great friend of Paderewski, the wizard of the ivory keys, and he said to me, "Did you ever realize how it is possible for Paderewski to swarm up and down those flights and every note be even in tone, and yet distinct from each other ? How he can race the key board with a crescendo of music, and repeat it like a whisper, but every note is distinct and event It is because he has powerful fingers. They are like steel cables, and his grasp is like a vice." Well, I figured my friend ought to know, for he is a very powerful man himself and an ardent exerciser. I was not surprised to hear that. It seemed logical in Paderewski's case. But I have seen many various demonstrations of finger strength, and each feat is the exercise that made the fingers so capable when the feat was shown. Therefore, a person has a pretty wide range of instruction from which they can glean many things that are very valuable in helping them to acquire finger strength.

So far as lifting weights with the fingers goes, I believe that Warren Lincoln Travis is the best man in the world. He certainly is the best that I ever met, in raising weights off the floor with the aid of his fingers. I have seen him make several big lifts with two fingers, but the best he ever did was the time he celebrated his fiftieth birthday, when he raised the terrific weight of eight hundred and eighty-one and one-half pounds, using just one finger of each hand. I was the referee on that occasion, and was proud to see Travis raise the world's record so high. On the one finger lift he has done around five hundred and sixty pounds, while John Pagano has also raised over five hundred pounds with one finger. The lift is not made with the bare finger, as you are no doubt aware. The finger could not grasp the object to lift it. The middle finger is used, and on it the lifter fits an iron eye that has a hook attached, which grabs the object to be lifted. It is necessary that the eye should fit tightly upon the finger up at the first joint, as close to the knuckle of the hand as possible, as the finger is crooked, the eye locks thereon. Just the same it has to be raised off the floor, and that takes power. The ligament of that finger becomes very thick. In some cases, I have seen it become so thick that it made the finger crooked. A few years ago I met an old Swedish lifter who had quit the profession, but in his day was claimed to be a great finger lifter. I remember quite well that the middle finger of his right hand was almost twice as large as any of his other fingers, just from practicing that lift.

A splendid pastime to test your finger strength, and at the same time build it, is finger pulling. You lock your middle finger with that of your opponent's at the first joint near the hand, then you both pull, and the finger that is first straightened out, loses the pull. Teddy Mack has very strong fingers. On one occasion he and I locked fingers together and resisted the pull of ten men, trying to get us apart, five on each side.

I once had a husky young bar bell user call on me, and among some of the stunts that he did was making a handstand on all fingers, and finally making a perfect stand using only two fingers and the thumbs of each hand. I have seen John Y. Smith, the famous Boston strongman, do the same feat when he was in his sixtieth year. However, Professor Paulinetti told me he knew a professional balancer who actually made a hand stand using only the index finger and the thumb of each hand.

Among other clever demonstrations of finger strength, that I had the pleasure of witnessing, was a feat by my pupil Philippe Fournier, of Montreal. At the Joffre Cafe where he, Giroux, and the famous Parisian lifter, Cadine trained when in Montreal, was an old solid type bar bell that weighed two. hundred and fifteen pounds, and the bar was one and a quarter inches in diameter. By employing just the middle finger of each hand, Fournier made a two hands Clean and Jerk with this bell, which completely stumped the giant Giroux and the clever French lifter, Cadine. It was a terrific feat and I doubt if there is a man living who can duplicate it. Although' Fournier only weighs one hundred and fifty-four pounds, he is prodigiously strong, and has exceptionally strong fingers. I have seen him take a large size horseshoe nail, and with the bare fingers of his hands, twist it into spirals like a corkscrew. Another very interesting stunt I saw him do was to place the back of his hand upon a chair, and let the heaviest man present place his thumb upon the first joint of his middle finger; then he told him to force down with all his weight and might, but it was useless. Fournier actually curled that one joint of the finger where all the weight was sustained, without even moving the hand or the other fingers. Despite all the efforts of the man to keep that finger pressed down, Fournier lifted him up, and it is claimed no man has ever been successful in holding the finger down. I remember this feat among the most remarkable, for finger strength, that I ever saw. In wrist turning also Fournier is very powerful; he actually makes most of his living this way, backing himself against all comers without a single defeat so far, being registered against him.

A feat of finger strength I have often seen practiced with a billiard cue, is to take the point of the cue and place it just under the index finger, with the weight of the cue supported upon the back of the other fingers. The feat is to press against the tip of the cue so that the full length of it lies in a straight line with the back of the hand. I once heard of a man thus holding out three, but I did not see him do it. However, the information was reliable and surely was a real feat of finger strength. Another feat is to gather the tips of as many billiard cues as you are able, within the grasp of the fingers of one hand only, and hold them out at arms' length, level with the shoulders. Six is the most I ever heard of being correctly handled in this manner. It is a much more difficult feat than a person imagines. Just try one for a start, and then see how terribly awkward two is. Each additional one makes the feat still more difficult.

Coin bending and breaking is another test for finger strength, but it is a rare thing to see such a stunt performed. John Marx and Albert Shakesby are the only two I ever saw that could break them, and they were not new coins either. I know many others claim to have done this, but I am dubious of most of them unless I personally see them break my own coins, as in the two cases mentioned.

Charles Vanstittart, the famous English athlete of a decade ago who was famed as the man with the iron grip, could wrap up plates of pewter, like paper, with only the use of his fingers. He was also capable of tearing a brand new tennis ball into pieces with his finger strength. He was a man endowed with genuine power, and he was above any shady practices.

To see a man take something in his hands and crush it, tear or lift, has always had a fascinating influence over everybody. For some unknown reason, such feats seem to grip the layman with greater interest than great bodily feats of strength.

Some time ago, a certain strong man was boosted for his great ability to lift fifty pound plates of iron by the edge with his finger strength, and walk away with one in each hand. I know of scores who can duplicate the feat, many of whom are just light men. I have seen several different athletes who were capable of snatching one in each hand overhead, both at the same time. Right here in Philadelphia, I can place my hands on two amateur bar bell men who can raise seventy-five pound plates off the floor, gripping .them by the edge with their fingers only. It is a mighty task and takes a powerful grip.

One time when Joe Nordquest was in Philadelphia, he and Teddy Mack were resting on chairs among the weights, when Joe reached down and grasped a thick fifty pound plate by the edge and curled it to the shoulder as pretty as a picture. Completely effortless. Wouldn't you feel you were strong if you could do that?

A feat that is more difficult than picking up a fifty pound plate, is to span with the hand the bottom face of a fifty pound block weight and raise it off the ground. It is very hard to get hold of; practically only the tips of the fingers are able to take a hold, with the thumb. Robert Ruckstool is very efficient at this stunt, and his hand is not extra long, but he does it neatly. Here is another very difficult feat which I unexpectedly ran up against some years ago. I was calling on a very well known strong man, and he told me he was going to introduce me to a German athlete who was very strong. I was glad to meet him, and quite naturally we got talking about strength, and the first thing I knew was that this son of Anan brought forward a round ball of iron and asked me to lift it. Personally I don't think a man should expect another to equal him on a feat which he had specialized upon for years and condemn him if he fails. I am always willing to try anything whether I fail or not, but I prefer men should test their merits on a matter of stunts, rather than hold to their specialty. This man was very boastful and loud in his belief that I could not lift the ball of iron. I told him I would not be surprised if I failed, as the ball was very large for my hand and finger, while the other man had a much larger hand. Three times he failed to raise it, but to my surprise and to his consternation, I lifted it on the second attempt.

I have found that anything that has a very large diameter should not be gripped too tightly. If this is done, the object is forced out of the hand. A grip that is inclined to be loose is the best. If you ever watch a manipulator of coins or billiard balls work, notice how easily he seems to hold them within his fingers.

A little further back, I was talking of lifting plates of iron by the edges. If you want something a little more of a teaser than a fifty pound plate, just take two twenty-five pound plates with beveled edges, and stand them on their edge side by side; then span the two with the hand and raise them. It is a little more catchy, as the plates slip against each other, and with the beveled edges they help to neutralize your finger grip.

Chinning the bar with the fingers is a test you do not see performed every day. I have seen Charles Schaffer chin himself perfectly three times with one finger. I have seen him stand between two boards that supported a floor, and catch hold of the joist between the thumb and fingers of each hand. Hanging thus, he never had any difficulty in chinning himself. Later I saw him walk between the two joists, hanging in the manner he chinned himself. He would chin himself hanging on one joist with the palms of the hands facing him; although the walk along is much more difficult.

When I get thinking about finger strength used in chinning, I always remember the remarkable feat performed by Professor Schmidt. I never saw any one who could duplicate it, or ever hold their bodyweight for a fraction of a second in the manner I am going to explain. He would tie a length of chain on a horizontal bar, just high enough overhead so that he could reach up and grasp it. Now I want you to get this right so you will better appreciate the feat. The links in the chain were not the long wide links that allowed you to hook your finger in them. They were links that were too small to allow any such hold. Well, Schmidt would take hold of the last link with only his index finger and thumb, in much the same way that you would hold a pencil lengthwise between your index finger and thumb. With only this slight catch, the professor would positively chin himself and hold himself chinned. He weighs about one hundred and twenty-five pounds, but I have seen some of the cleverest finger chinners in existence hopelessly fail at this test. It is a feat that you do not have to attempt to duplicate to realize its enormity. Your imagination will explain it sufficiently.

I once saw a sailor take a cocoanut and crush it to pieces between the palms of his hand, by interlacing his fingers. The feat is equally an arm feat, but if his fingers were not strong, they would have pulled apart under the great pressure.

Lock your middle fingers together and allow some of your friends to try and pull you apart. See how much resistance you can withstand in this manner. It is a good test and helps to make a good exhibition feat.

Talking about feats with an anvil reminds me of a particular feat that I performed impromptu which takes a great amount of confidence as well as strength. It happened at one of the times that I picked up an anvil by the horn in a smithy shop, and after that stunt I pressed the anvil to arms' length by lying it on its broadside upon the flat of my hand, which is not as easy as it sounds. After I had done this I put the anvil on the floor on its base. We began to talk about various anvil feats being so difficult because of its awkward unbalanced construction. One man remarked that it would be some stunt to balance the anvil on the hand upside down. That meant the face would rest on the hand and the heavy wide base on top. Somehow I conceived the notion I could do it, and accordingly I took hold of the face with my right hand, and with the help of the left arm got the weight to the shoulder. Despite the wide base and the bad balance caused by same and the horn, I not only succeeded in balancing the anvil by its face, but pressed it to arms' length, to the amazement of all. I have done it many times since, and for this volume I performed the same feat, thinking it might interest my readers. The anvil weighed one hundred sixty-eight pounds.

Now you may think that these two feats have nothing to do with finger strength. Well it has, and a great deal. In the first feat where the anvil lies broadside upon the hand, the great pressure of the concaved side forces the hand back tremendously. If you have not the finger strength to resist the pressure, the hand will be forced too far backwards and the feat made impossible. In the last described feat, only the thumb and the ends of the fingers span the anvil's face and it is these slight catches that enabled me to control the balance and keep the anvil perpendicular throughout the feat.

The Canadian lifters have a feat in which finger strength is very important. In one way, they see who can carry the heaviest dumb-bell the farthest, in each hand, before the weight pulls out of the fingers. Another way, a bar bell is lifted, like in the two hands dead lift, and the walker tries how far he can walk forwards —not sideways—with the bar bell in his hands. It is difficult to walk this way, as the bar bell is in the way of the forward leg movement. I saw Arthur Giroux in a contest, walk fifteen feet with a bar bell weighing 657 pounds, before his fingers were straightened. Giroux and Gorner would make a great pair in such a contest, as both have powerful hands and fingers, and have so far proven themselves the greatest men in the world on such feats of strength.

Get a bunch of your fellow exercise fans together, and try some of these stunts. You will get fun and profit from them, and they help to break up the monotony that might exist in constant ordinary exercise training. You will never miss the time spent this way. It is an interesting play that keeps your enthusiasm alive, and will have a valuable influence upon the size and strength of your forearm.

CHAPTER X
FAMOUS MEN OF MIGHT AND MUSCLE

To me the rim of the horizon was always full of mystery, and as maturity claimed me, I longed eagerly to solve its hidden meanings for myself. It seems but yesterday that I heard my mother croon, "A Wednesday babe wanders far away," and I, in my childish faith, would ask her what I would be when I grew to be a man. My star of destiny rose at birth on the wanderers* trail, a path I followed for so many years. Now. as I look back, I can see in the gleam of bivouac and camp fire, on veldt and prairie, little gatherings of restless, wistful men. I loved to listen to the lives of others as they lived their battles over in the tales they told. 1 he lumberjack s shanty, the soldier s bivouac and the sailor's galley, each is a sacred spot, and so is the little club room o5 the gym. where the strong men have gathered for years and then passed on, leaving their appointed place to be filled by others of a younger generation. Does history repeat itself? I do not know; it always seems new to me. However, we all like to listen to it. The audience may be the same, drawn by a common appeal that is handed down. To us, the call of the strong man, the man of iron, is the spark that ignites our enthusiasm, We are all interested in the deeds of the modern strong man, but the deeds of the mighty men who in other days wielded Vulcan's rod, still claim our greater attention. So it will always be. The man of today will be the hero of tomorrow. His deeds will remain to thrill others, just as the deeds of the mighty iron men of a past decade continue to thrill us. So, gather around comrades, old and young, while I tell you some of the stories of men of might and muscle, I have known and heard of, and may my recitals interest you as much as the telling interests me.

I am not going to stick to any set form. I am just going to narrate to you the incidents as they come to my mind, in my own rambling style, to let you glimpse some of the characteristics of the famous strong men, their personality and good fellowship. So you can smile more steadfastly, in the realization of the fact that once a man is strong, he is always strong, no matter where you place him. Looking into his life we will see the evidence of his mighty strength in many difficult phases. No man can say a man is really strong unless his strength will prove itself under all circumstances. Our common sense knows that. Place any other man in the same circumstances I shall narrate and he would prove himself a physical pigmy. The strongman who obtained his strength from bar bell training, and who took to tossing iron for his particular sport, is still the monarch of strength athletes. No other method can give the same thews, or convey the same inspiring message to those who seek the domain of health and strength. Years ago, after the French Canadian giant, Louis Cyr, had forsaken the stage to take charge of his saloon in Montreal, thousands of his admirers continued to pay homage to him. They constantly patronized his saloon so they could claim friendship with this iron king. They listened to him tell his stories, but always with a hope and a watchful eye to see him perform some feat which to him was common-place, but to others impossible. It was no uncommon sight to see Louis carry a huge cask of beer off the drayman's wagon on his one shoulder. What was a three hundred and twenty pound cask to him, even if it was terribly awkward to handle. He could grasp it by the chines and lift it from the wagon to the pavement, and then toss it on one shoulder, or throw it back on the truck, according to the need, without registering any sign of exertion. It was all in a day's work to him, but one feat he often performed to draw patronage as a part of his business routine. Yet, he always performed it in an offhand way, that made him appear to be indifferent to any effect the feat had upon the spectators. They still talk about it in the old haunts, and it is a story worth telling.

Cyr would be reclining on the serving side of the bar and while he was in the midst of his conversation with his patrons, he would be approached by his wife dressed to go shopping. With the interrogative "Louis," she would announce her presence. Knowing what she wanted, the ponderous giant would neither withdraw his gaze or stop in his speech, but would lower his right hand in a nonchalant fashion, upon which his wife would sit. As gently as a child he would lift her over the counter, and as gently deposit her on the other side without a break in his speech. Madam would be examining her purse during the unusual journey and would then pass on as calmly as though she had made the trip in a modern elevator. Showmanship par-excellence was exhibited by both in this extraordinary feat, but can you imagine the amount of strength that was involved ? Although she did not weigh much over a hundred pounds, yet it meant that he curled her weight on the flat of his hand, and passed her over the counter in the manner of a hold-out and with no visible effort. It was a terrific feat of strength, which when performed, was a source of delight to all who witnessed it.

It is a well known fact that Louis was an enormous gourmand, and his old show partner, Horace Barre, who retired a few years before Cyr, could keep him company at any of his feasts. These orgies were the cause of the death of both men. Many claim that the Bourgeaux jailor was stronger than Cyr, but it is hard to say, as both were Goliaths in strength. One of the outstanding feats of Barre's career, and one which he performed on three occasions, was that of walking the length of the gymnasium with a bar bell that weighed twelve hundred and seventy pounds on his shoulders. Twice he carried the weight in Montreal and once he duplicated the feat in Professor Attila's gymnasium in New York. Some time ago I was talking to the wife of the late professor, and we naturally fell to discussing Louis Cyr and Horace Barre. Madam Attila remembered quite well when the huge French Canadian made the astounding lift. We laughed as we recalled the quaint superstitions that obsessed poor Barre. If things were not just so, you might as well try to move the Woolworth Building, as poor superstitious Horace. He was full of signs and omens, and was forever crossing himself. Both he and Louis were good, honest hearted souls. Their life requirements were simple and they always had a smile for every one; I never heard of either having any enemies.

Carl Moerke, reminds me of Cyr, in build, except that Cyr was a much bigger man. Carl is only five feet two inches and weighs two hundred and twenty pounds, but his bulk for his height can be compared with Cyr's. Moerke is also tremendously strong. If you want to give yourself an idea of what his capabilities are, ask yourself what you could do with one of the steel rails that lie on a railway track. Perhaps you do not know much about them, but the next time you see the men laying railroad rails, see how many men it takes to carry one. A long rail weighs about one thousand pounds. On one occasion, Moerke carried one of these rails in his hands, with the rail balanced across his abdomen, to its resting place on the track. No wonder he can do a deep knee bend with nearly six hundred pounds. When he was visiting me, I saw him snatch a bar bell of one hundred and sixty pounds overhead with one finger. Not off the floor as you might imagine. First he stood erect with the weight hanging at arms' length on his finger; then with a quick knee bend he took the weight to arms' length overhead. He is not lacking in the real stuff, and I have often had the pleasure of seeing this for myself; neither is his fellow country man and old opponent Henry Steinborn.

One time I met four German athletes who had been interned in the same prison camp as Henry, in Australia. They told me that for a weight they had sawed a tree trunk in two and connected the two pieces together with a long rod. That was their bar bell, and such as you can imagine was some weapon. In that prison camp there were thirty men who could lift three hundred pounds overhead, which was the weight of this improvised bar bell. Some days only about four could lift it. For a while they could not imagine what was wrong, until one day Henry got stumped. He became sore and after a great fight he got the weight overhead. Out of curiosity they weighed it, and found that instead of weighing three hundred pounds, it weighed three hundred and seventy-five pounds. It started them guessing. Then they got the answer. It had rained incessantly for two or three days and the timber had become water-logged, and a few days later when it had dried out, it weighed three hundred pounds as before. However, whenever there was a heavy dew or a shower, the wood absorbed it, which was the reason why the majority were so often stuck. Henry claims that was what made him a lifter, although the method of progression was not the sort that most of us would care much about. Yet, it must have been funny to see Henry get sore at his bell.

Talking about getting sore, can you imagine the even-tempered Warren Lincoln Travis getting sore? He did once. He was giving an exhibition down in New England, and at the entrance of the show he had his diamond belt and some other trophies on display. He had hired a man to watch them, but Warren forgot to hire somebody else to watch the watcher. The result was, the caretaker of the trophies beat it with the whole outfit, which is worth a snug fortune. Did Warren camp on that guy's trail? OH! boy, he didn't wait for a train. The spirit of Achilles was in his heels, and he was travelling faster than any train. But, the best Travis could do was to locate the pawn shop where the smart boy had hocked the goods. Warren wept for joy when he grabbed his cherished possessions, but the thief got away. Lucky for him, for if Travis had ever got his hands on him, it would have been the parting of the ways, as Warren would have distributed him to the four winds. However, Warren still remembers it and is willing to laugh with you over the escapade.

The only times Apollon, the French giant, could ever be made to show what he could really do, were when he was sore. In his act he used to appear in a prison scene. It was an epic. The stage was shrouded in darkness with the back curtain reflecting the fitful lights of a stormy night. The pale moon appeared from behind a cloudy crest, as it silhouetted the prison in grim foreboding lines. Clearly, the high railings cast their shadows; then suddenly a tall figure wrapped in a long cloak which failed to conceal the powerful lines beneath rushed from the cover of the prison walls and flung himself at the heavy iron rails which separated him from freedom. Grasping a rail in each hand, he pulled and tugged until they were forced wide apart to form an aperture through which he leaped to the front of the stage, as the music crashed into a triumphant march, and the lights went on revealing the Herculean features of Apollon, the idol of France. After each performance, the railings had to be taken to the blacksmith shop to be straightened. One of these excursions almost proved disastrous to our hero. The blacksmith, thinking he was doing Apollon a good turn, thought he would see how hard he could temper the rails to prevent them from further bending. He was only too successful. That evening Apollon came on to do his stuff, but to his surprise the bars refused to yield. Now this big son of Gaul was always considered lazy, and when he married, as usual, the law of opposites prevailed. He won for himself a very small bride, but what she lacked in size she certainly possessed in temper; and by all accounts, Madame was the real Omphale to this Hercules. Seeing him make no impression on the bars, she thought he had developed another of his lazy spells, and from the wings she stamped her tiny feet and tongue-lashed

143

her bigger half to make him exert himself. Struggling with all his might, he was only able to spread the rails wide enough to squeeze himself through. Utterly played out, he was unable to continue with his act and was obliged to leave the stage. His ponderous arms had swollen inches larger with the great exertion, until they resembled columns of twisted steel. It would have been an impossible task for another, and I feel that none of the iron twisters of the present time would have made the slightest impression on the bars that evening. This giant was idolized for many years in France and is considered by the French one of the greatest of strong men that ever lived, which I do not doubt. His right name is Louis Uni, and he commenced lifting weights in a circus when only a very young boy. At the present time he is about sixty-five years of age, but unfortunately in 1913 he was badly injured in his act pulling against two automobiles, and this injury afterwards made him a cripple. He was reported to have been killed, but it was later found that he was living in retirement in Paris, where he now is. Some claim the feat was not genuine, as they do not believe it possible to pull against an automobile, but they are mistaken; for if the driver shifts quickly into high gear to start the machine, a powerful man can stall the car. The stronger a man is, the longer he can sustain the pull, and he is Capable of handling a heavier machine. Probably what happened was one of the drivers went into low gear and stayed there, which was worse than if both had gone into low gear. Apollon was fifty-three when this happened and crippled as he is today, at sixty-five, he could make a lot of them take a back seat, just like George Hackenschmidt did in Vienna a couple of years ago. Here was a man who radiated a personality very different from that possessed by most strong men. He loved to dress well and was always a model of fashion. When he broke Sandow's One Arm Press record, he took more pride in the faultlessly tailored pair of pants that his patron solemnly presented him, in view of the audience, than in the expensive gold medal given him to commemorate his splendid lift. It was the way George disposed of his opponents when wrestling, that amused everybody. His colossal strength enabled him to pitch his adversaries around, like baseballs. At the time he was going strongest, the song of the day was "In the Shade of the Old Apple Tree." Some bright boy composed a parody on it, which my friends used to always make me sing as my contribution at any of the athletic feasts I attended. It went like this, "When Hackenschmidt grappled with me, he pulled like the roots of a tree. He gave me a punch, where I just had my lunch, and he mixed up my dinner and tea. Well I had no choice, don't you see, 'cos he had the half nelson on me. And he made such a wreck, at the back of my neck, that he punctured my old apple tree." Those were the happy days, when life seemed to be full of laughter and happiness.

At the same time, Arthur Saxon was dazzling the world with his matchless strength, and when I hear that it is claimed that the Bent Press was a trick lift, I get a wonderful laugh. Particularly, when they try to measure Arthur's strength by that lift. When any one claims that Saxon was not mighty, he only proves his own ignorance. Take the Bent Press, his specialty from him, and set? what he could do. For instance, whoever lifted his sack of flour? Nobody. Wherever he went, the finest huskies tried their best, but no matter how they tried, their strength was never equal to the task. But look how Saxon handled it. He certainly employed no elaborate method to lift it. To my knowledge he used a perfectly natural method that anybody who tried could use, but his method of lifting the sack of flour was entirely hopeless for others to try. Simply straddling the three hundred and twenty pound sack of flour he interlaced his fingers beneath the center, and with one heave, he had the bulky object to his chest, changing his grip as the sack arrived at the shoulders. Then overhead it went. The jolly miller was just as useless on that stunt as the store clerk, Shape, size or balance of an object never seemed to bother Saxon. Why look at the way he handled that barrel of beer, which weighed over three hundred and ten pounds. Grasping it by the chines, he could tear it off the ground to arms' length overhead and hold it there, despite the roll of the beer which made it difficult to keep the balance. I never heard of a drayman,—who is always good at handling kegs and barrels—handling anything like the weight contained in that cask of beer in such a manner, and Saxon gave everyone the same chance. If they could lift it, they could have it, but like the sack of flour, no one ever got it. Even more marvelous was the manner in which he snatched the plank overhead. This plank of wood weighed one hundred and eighty pounds. He would stand it on its two-inch edge holding it with only the grip of his fingers and thumb. In one movement, it went aloft. Just you try to lift a two-inch plank, weighing one hundred and eighty pounds, off the floor, and you will be trying something. These are feats which the miller, drayman and lumberman should be good at, as they are their specialties, but none ever came forward to duplicate the feats, and I never heard of any who could. I have seen some very strong men among these three groups, and have seen them do some wonderfully good stuff; yet the best of them have suffered badly by comparison with a real strong man. He can beat them all in nearly every test he is put up against.

Just look at John Marx. There was another powerful man. No matter where you put him, he was strong. The way he could bend and break horse shoes was remarkable. One feat he did for some time, which always made a great impression on the people, was to break a chain with a blow of his hand. The way he did it was to stretch tight between two uprights a length of trace chain, and with a quick downward blow of his fist, he snapped it in two. The little finger of his right hand was broken quite often by this stunt.

Finally he gave it up for that reason. He had a very impressive figure when dressed, and he knew it. Although he was never conceited about it, he used his appearance as a business attraction, just as Joe Coryn of Pittsburgh did years ago. You would always see John wearing a Prince Albert suit with a high hat and carrying a gold headed walking stick in his hand. Thus attired, he would stroll majestically along the streets. As he walked, everybody would turn to watch him. The wide back, deep chest, massive shoulders, powerful neck, and the flat waist, made him an imposing sight. One time, in one of the cities where he was showing, he was strolling along the main street, when he approached a group of young fellows who were a little the worse for drink, and who apparently were familiar with John by sight. One of the group evidently wanting to show off began to strut in front of John, regally puffing on an imaginary cigar, and holding a stick of wood in his other hand to imitate the gold headed stick that Marx carried. In an arrogant voice the drunken swaggerer bawled out, "Make way for the great John Marx, I am coming." About this time John had caught up with the would- be clown, and as though oblivious to his existence as a human being, he grasped him by the seat of the pants and lifted him high off his feet, like an object to be removed. With no effort John held him thus, and continued his walk a few steps. Then he dropped the now badly scared youth into a rubbish cart that was parked on the side of the road. So easily and so casually did the big athlete handle the weight of the other man that his friends just gasped. John paid no more attention to them than he would have shown them if the incident had never happened.

This little chastisement reminds me of another correction in behavior that was meted out by Emile De Riaz, the elder brother of the famous Maurice De Riaz. I might say that Emile was equally famous and has some fine records to his name, but he did not continue as long as a professional athlete as Maurice. He got married and settled down to keep a saloon in Paris that was very popular with both athletes and laymen. One drink Emile refused to keep, and that was absinthe. Rather an unusual procedure for a French saloon, but Emile being a Swiss never got accustomed to recognize this as a necessary beverage, as most French people do. Madame De Riaz was a very beautiful woman, and one day as she was attending the wants of the patrons, while her husband was working in the cellar, a loud speaking man, evidently under the influence of absinthe, seated himself at a table. He began to call for absinthe, and when Madame informed him that they did not serve it, he became very objectionable in his remarks. Seeing that he would neither keep quiet nor go out, Madame rang a bell for Emile, who quickly appeared. Quietly looking in at the door, he saw the cause of the trouble and without a word he turned on his heels, appearing shortly with a hammer and nail in his hands. Without paying any attention to the brawler, Emile took a chair and stood on it as he drove the nail in the wall, high up, but immediately over the head of the man who was still making himself obnoxious. This done, Emile reached down and grabbed his man by the coat collar and with a snap he jerked him off the seat, and before any one realized what had happened, the brawler was suspended from the nail by the coat collar. There Emile left him to kick out of his evil temper. When he was lowered to the ground it was as a strictly reformed man, who gladly and humbly apologized to Madame. The general rule was to throw such people out into the gutter, but Emile found a better way. Still his method needed a strong man to be able to use it.

Not long ago, a press photographer showed me a picture of a strong man carrying a large rowboat on his shoulders. He was walking with his burden down the beach to the sea and continued his walk until the boat with its occupant floated off his shoulder. The entire weight was over four hundred pounds, and a boat is a very hard object to handle. When I gazed upon the face of the man, I was not surprised as I recognized Henry Steinborn.

Sometimes, more than others, I feel that the world loves a strong man just as much as a man glories in his own strength. Life without it loses all its value, and we would miss a lot of the thrills that go with strength. Even though it is great to watch a really strong man work, it is much greater to be able to do some of the things yourself.

One of the greatest impressions of my life came, like most of them, quite unexpectedly. I was standing in a little railroad junction in the North of England, where I had to make a connection. It was a beautiful spot tucked away in a valley that bloomed with variegated nature. I had been absorbed examining the ruins of an ancient abbey, and the remains of the old Roman wall that ran partly through the valley. Turning from them, I saw sitting upon the seat on the platform, an enormously proportioned man. He had the shoulders of Hercules and limbs of a great thickness that showed their size through his clothes. As I gazed at him, he rose to face me, and across his majestic breast in three rows were numerous medals. I was in the presence of Albert Shakesby, who was then widely known as the Athlete Evangelist. I had long been curious to meet him, for since I had been up in the north, many had passed the remark that we looked much alike, although he was built on a scale about twice the size of myself. I know the name will mean nothing to you, but let me tell you that if there ever was a man in the world who represented strength of mind, body and character, it was Albert Shakesby. His extraordinary strength, like the strength of the biblical Samson, was a boon to him and a godsend to many. He holds the honored record of saving more lives from death,—drowning, accidents, etc.—than any other man. He could do anything, swim, box, wrestle, lift weights, sprint, cycle, or anything you can mention, and he was a topnotcher at them all. He was one of the few men that Britain had who could make Hackenschmidt work to throw him. He forsook the athletic profession aft(r he had embraced religion. Stripped, he weighed around two hundred and twenty-five pounds and was a mass of muscle. He and John Marx were the only two men who ever actually bent and broke a coin of mine in two, in my presence. Shakesby never cared to do such things, but I insisted so strongly, because I wanted to retain something as a souvenir of our meeting. Not a great while before our meeting, he had sustained a very serious accident while saving a life at a fire. He just happened to be in the vicinity of the fire and became one of the many spectators. The fire spread over the building very rapidly, and it was believed that everybody was out, but to the horror of the watchers, a form appeared at one of the windows on the third floor. The flames drove the trapped man out on the window ledge, where he missed his footing and came hurtling down head first. Like a flash, Shakesby jumped forward and caught the man by the head in cupped hands, heaving upwards with all his might, which broke the fall and saved the man from serious injury. Just pause a moment and think what an enormous amount of strength was required for this life-saving feat. As you know, it is hard enough to withstand the impact of a body from the distance of our height; then what must have been the impact of this man's bodyweight from the height of three stories. Every foot of the way his poundage would increase with the speed of the fall. But Shakesby was powerful enough to withstand the shock. At one time he had a gymnasium, and he said that when he saw the man fall, immediately he thought of the method employed by instructors to put falling pupils on their feet. This is done by heaving up on the head.

He was one of the very few men I ever saw who could take a two hundred pound dumb-bell off the floor clean to the shoulder and put it overhead without moving the feet, which were held military style with heels together. He held numerous honors from the Royal Humane Society for his life-saving feats and was a monument of inspiration to the cause of body culture. He was great at tearing decks of cards, but I do not remember how many he could tear. In this feat the best man I ever heard of was Al Treloar. Some of the old-timers will remember him as the man who won one of the early MacFadden posing contests. That must have been more than twenty years ago. I remember seeing his picture posed as "Sin" on the cover page of Physical Culture. It struck me as being very beautiful. Treloar could tear four decks of cards all at once. A year ago Al had charge of some tumblers from Los Angeles, where he has been instructing for years now. He had brought them east to compete and stopped in to see me. The only thing he regretted was that I did not have enough card decks handy to show me that he was as efficient today as he was twenty-five years ago. He has great hand strength, and like all good men is very unassuming.

I have written quite a bit about hand strength, but what would you think of a man who had such arm strength that when he wrapped his arms around the body, he could crush the ribs in. There was such a man. He was a French provincial wrestler and strong man, whose name unfortunately has slipped my memory. They used to tell a story, that one time when he was with a carnival wrestling, he got enraged at his opponent who was as elusive as an eel. In one of the sorties he caught his adversary around the body and swept him off his feet. He crushed him so terribly with his arms that the blood gushed from his mouth and the man died. The wrestler had remarkable pectoral and arm development, and he was a marvel at raising weights from the crucifix position lying on the floor. I was told that he had raised one hundred pounds in each hand that way. It was a terrific feat, but he surely looked capable of doing it. This reminds me of a feat I saw Vanbruch, a Dutch strong man, perform when I was in Amsterdam. We had all been doing stunts with a flat ring weight that weighed fifty-six pounds, and among the stunts we tried was holding the weight out level with the shoulders by the ring. We all succeeded, as this is not much of a feat. Two men held it out with their little finger, then we quit, having done all the stunts we knew. During all the time, Vanbruch had merely been a spectator, and as we concluded, he stepped forward. He turned the weight over, ring down and spanned the flat side with one hand, only his fingers holding the weight. In this manner he held the weight out at arms' length, level with the shoulder, retaining the grip on the weight until he lowered his arm to place the ring weight on the floor. Needless to say this stunt stopped us all. I doubt if Empian, the old time famous French "muscle out" champion, could have done it. Since that time, I have often mentioned it to various strong men I have encountered, but none have ever been successful in my sight.

It used to be that when we all got together, an impromptu elimination tournament commenced, and I have seen many surprising feats performed at such times. The men, whose names are most familiar to us, are not always the supreme beings. There are many strong men who are practically never heard of, who just try out their strength for pastime, but I never knew one who did not train with bar-bells, or whose daily occupation did not involve work similar to lifting weights.

I do not suppose many of my readers will remember the Italian who called himself the original Milo. He had a fine physique, and one of his feats was to balance a piano upon his chin while a young lady assistant played a tune. Of course, the piano was not nearly as heavy as the ordinary piano, but at the lightest and with a person attached to it, it stands as an astounding feat of both skill and strength. Sometimes I find it very hard to estimate the strength of some men, for they seem to be capable of performing such astonishing feats, that no matter how you figure they accomplished it, the feat remains a near miracle. Veritable giants of strength in action, but dressed on the streets, they would not impress the ordinary person as being such producers. There are a few exceptions, but the majority of men I can recall to mind, never showed their quality in their ordinary street attire; giants in strength, but seldom in stature. As a matter of fact, few giants have ever been recorded as being strong. The only one I can vouch for is Angus McAskill of Nova Scotia. This human dinosaur stood seven feet nine inches high, and weighed five hundred and sixty pounds. It is stated that his normal chest measurement was eighty inches. They tell some very remarkable tales about some of the feats he performed, which sound much like a chapter from the pages of the "Arabian Nights." Still, when you stop and figure out on a mathematical scale, the leverage his height gave him, with the weight he had, he must have been quite capable. One or two of his feats which are often talked about have been done by men two feet shorter than he, and two hundred and sixty pounds lighter. We can safely say that a boy standing four feet nine inches and weighing one hundred pounds is, if anything, heavy for his height, and we know that a man who stands five feet and nine inches, and strips at around two hundred is a mighty fine type of a man. Allowing one hundred pounds for each foot over four feet nine inches, we have a pretty fair standard, which makes McAskill one hundred and sixty pounds overweight for his height. Yet, this extra weight can be better distributed over seven feet nine inches, than an extra one hundred can be, over the body of a man of five feet nine inches. At the same time, we have had powerful men with that much excess weight. To mention two, Cyr and Barre, make a fair comparison. This would bring McAskill in the class of super-men, like the men just mentioned. He was prodigiously strong beyond a doubt, and while it is said he did not like work, yet he loved to exhibit his great strength. The Queen of England heard of this man and expressed the doubt that such a being lived. In order to satisfy her majesty, McAskill journeyed to England and performed before the Queen, who presented him with a handsome gift in gold. He used to travel in a circus, and when showing in Boston he made a wager that he could lift a certain anchor which weighed twenty-two hundred and fifty pounds to his shoulder. He is credited with not only lifting the anchor to the shoulder, but also with fifteen fathoms of the chain dragging, he walked with his burden for one hundred yards, from the end of the wharf to Atlantic Avenue. Later in life, he quit the circus to keep a store in Halifax, and natives of that city have often told me that when any person asked for a pound of tea, he just grabbed a hand full out of the sack and wrapped it up. The length of his hand was twelve inches and it was six inches wide. It is said that his handful of tea or sugar weighed a good pound. His footwear was size eighteen. No doubt he would have made a great wrestler, with such sized feet. All he would have to do would be to step on his man and with that five hundred and sixty pounds on top of that foot, it would be all over. Laying all jokes aside, if half they report of him is true, he must have been a marvel. I never paid a great deal of attention to the tales I heard until I met an old time weight lifter who was very reliable, and it was he who confirmed the anchor feat. If any of my readers happen to pass through Halifax, Nova Scotia, it would be worth their while to visit the museum where many of his relics are kept.

For many years the city of Vienna, in Austria, boasted of being the greatest center of strong men. At one time the ancient city could boast of having seventy known flourishing strong man clubs, but Munich is now running it hard for first place. Some claim that Munich is a greater center today than Vienna. Then again, there is Reval, in Russia, that can boast of a great number of powerful men.

In this city there is a special club to which no man is given membership unless he can qualify first by lifting in the Two Hands Clean and Jerk, at least three hundred pounds. With such a high standard of qualification, it is strange that we do not hear more of them. Perhaps the terrible condition of the country during the last few years accounts for their silence. Once a year in Europe, the strong men hold Stoerkefest. That is a gathering of strong men, past and present, who line up and parade the city in which the Stoerkefest is held. The people turn out for that, just as we in America turn out for a baseball game. Karl Swoboda still reigns as a great figure in the minds of the Europeans, even though he has dropped out of competition. It was the change of ruling on the different lifts that caused him to retire, but there is no doubt in my mind that in putting a weight over the head with two hands, anyway you can, Swoboda still reigns supreme. His actual achievements in competition, I will leave for another chapter. Here I just want to talk about strength in its other phases. Karl Swoboda is known as the Vienna butcher. In stature he is a huge man, weighing around three hundred pounds, with a nineteen-inch neck, biceps and calf. When he worked at slaughtering cattle, it was said that he could hold any beast powerless by the horns. I fully believe that, as I have seen it done by a huge slaughterman named Strides, who could play with three block weights in each hand as though they were only twenty-five pound dumb-bells. We can look all about us and see evidences of great feats of strength. All the time they are coming forward. At the present time the strength world has its eyes on Alzen of France, and Gorner of Germany, who look as though they are going to surpass them all. Yet, my mind still lingers around the huge LaVallee. Never will I forget the colossal power contained in that magnificent form. We talk about muscling out in the crucifix style, but where do any of them stand alongside of him. He was totally ignorant of the fact that he was making history when he stooped over and grasped in each hand by the short neck of the bags two, eighty-two pound cement sacks, and held out level with the shoulder, these heavy awkward objects that afforded such meager hand hold. And later he raised off the ground a bar-bell, loaded to nine hundred pounds. This was followed by picking up a crudely shaped dumb-bell that weighed a little over one hundred and sixty pounds, which he pressed overhead in a movement nearer to a one-hand Military Press than anything else. It was all impromptu lifting at that. He did not strip because he did not wish to exert himself. He was fully dressed in his working clothes with a sleeve vest. But look at the work he followed. It required all man power to execute it, and he knew he was very strong and took a joy in employing his powers. All day long he was lifting, lifting and lifting. Not with bar-bells or dumb-bells, of course, but more crude objects that answered the same purpose, which made him capable of handling heavy bar-bells. A man who is daily employed handling very heavy objects in various movements, is accumulating the power to enable him to do other things; just the same as the bar-bell fan training with more compact objects, over a series of exercises becomes able to demonstrate his powers on similar objects that require strength. Invariably the bar-bell man becomes more efficient than the vast majority of heavy manual workers, because he educates every muscle in his body. Better still, a person can be very weak and start training with bar-bells and get strong, but a man must be strong in the first place to be able to follow a heavy occupation. The most powerful men I ever knew realized the efficacy of exercise. It is the real goal winner. A very interesting proof of this was given me a few years ago. I was accosted by a long slim, pale, anemic young chap, who told me how deeply interested he was in strength. He said to me, "You know my weakness is the thorn in my soul. My dad is very strong and so is my brother, and they are always making me the butt. I can't work in the shop with them. I just have to stick in the office and that often gets me." Unconsciously, he clenched his fists and a flash shot through his eyes as he continued, "I'd give anything to be strong." I saw that there was a deeper motive than he had told me behind it. He was stung to the raw at being the family weakling. We talked for hours. Several months later he saw his chance. There was a heavy object which the father could not lift alone and he called to his strong son to come and help him. The weakling interrupted with the remark, "I'll lift that for you, dad," and to the amazement of father and brother, he lifted the object to the lathe. Conscious of the impression he had made, the former weakling effected an indifferent air as he walked away dusting off his hands with the parting cynicism, "When you get stuck, fellows, call on me." It was a transformation, and right now that young man can take his stand with many of the best where real man power is required.

There is a great joy in being strong, in being able to do the unexpected. One time two truck men were struggling unloading a huge barrel of oil. When they got it on the pavement, they left it reclining on its side, so it could be rolled, and as they rested a moment from their labors, the onlookers began to exclaim on the difficulty of handling such a heavy object and the impossibility of any one man handling it. At this last statement one of the truck men snorted with surprised disdain, "One man handle that! No danger, that kind of a man never was made." As though accepting a challenge, a stocky built spectator of medium height answered, "I believe I can handle it." All eyes turned on the speaker in a silence that spoke louder than words, as he stepped forward, and to their astonishment stood the barrel on end. This man was Teddy Mack. Another time he was called to the phone by a manufacturer of weights. This man said that he was up against a hard proposition. He had made a special bell but no one could lift it off the floor with

157

one hand. Why, they had no idea, as several well-known strong men were there unsuccessfully trying. Ted said he knew he could lift it before he saw it, and he informed them that he was coming right over. When he arrived he simply looked at the bell a few moments, listening to the other strong men talk. Suddenly he stooped over and said, "How's that?" and he immediately stood up with the weight in his one hand. Here is the reason for this instance. Mack was a strong man, who like a sprinter, tennis player, shot putter or hammer thrower, had the ability and knew how to apply it. Teddy Mack has unusual power in his arms and back, and knew how to use it.

When circuses were more plentiful than they are now, which dates back to before the time of auto transportation, all the trappings were heavily loaded on horse-drawn wagons, especially built for the purpose. In the season when the weather was bad, it was a frequent occurrence to get stuck on the bad roads. A wheel would drop in a big hole or the horses found the ruts too deep for them to pull the load through. At such times it was "get out and lift." All hands would have to get busy. Warren Lincoln Travis for years went with the circus, and with them he got plenty of impromptu workouts. When the circus help got stuck in helping a wagon out of a hole, or a rut, was the time when Travis would have to turn out and put his brawny back and powerful arms to the task. It was not uncommon to see him succeed where five or six men together had failed.

Strange how my mind is flitting around in this chapter, but as I finish reciting one incident, my mind snatches another from the panorama of mighty feats that crowd before me. As I thought of the surprise Travis always was to those circus huskies, I remember what a greater surprise Fournier has been to others, because he is so much smaller. One time an argument sprung up between Fournier and a big man who weighed more than three hundred pounds. The mountain of flesh snorted with disgust to think that there could be any comparison between himself and the little fellow. Finally one of Fournier's friends remarked, "Well, he can lift you, but you can't lift him," which was true. The big man weighed three hundred and fifteen pounds, and right there Fournier bent pressed him to arms' length overhead. Of course, it is easier to raise a man in this manner than a weight, when you get him to the shoulder, but still imagine the strength required to hold such a weight overhead. Another interesting feat performed by Fournier, who only weighed one hundred and fifty-four pounds at that time, was to toss a one hundred pound bar-bell in the air and catch it by the ball of one end upon the palm of one hand. Balancing it thus, on the hand, he pressed the bar-bell to arms' length overhead while preserving the balance. It makes a pretty snappy feat that will stop a lot of the best of them.

Joe Nordquest does a stunt of which very few would think him capable. Rarely do we hear of a heavy man able to do a one- hand stand. Joe not only does a one-hand stand, but in the disengaged hand he holds out a one hundred pound dumb-bell, with not a waver to his stand. For such a large man to do a one-hand stand is remarkable enough, but when he begins to juggle a hundred weight at the same time, it becomes a phenomenal feat.

Then there is the cross armed snatch of two hundred and thirty-one and a half pounds by Gorner, a feat which borders on the miraculous. As he takes hold of the handle bar of the weight, he crosses his arms so that the right hand grips where the left would ordinarily grip, and vice versa. In this cross armed fashion the weight is snatched perfectly to arms' length in one movement.

Such is man power. I could write books on the remarkable feats of strength I have seen performed, and these few incidents in this chapter are only a very few of the many feats I have seen performed by some of the many famous men of might and muscle. Reluctantly I must close this chapter to talk about other things, which I know will be full of interest to you.

CHAPTER XI
HOW A COLUMNAR NECK CREATES NERVE FORCE

In another chapter I made the remark that the calves were among the first things I looked over when making a physical survey of a body builder. If they lacked size and shapeliness, then his whole build was spoiled in my sight. If I want to find out how much physical force a man possesses, or is likely to possess in a dormant state, I look at his neck. That never fails to answer my question. In both man and the other male beasts, the neck has always been the true indication of the quality and quantity of his concentrated nerve power. A strong healthy man always has a powerful neck, and he always will have one.

When a man is sick or has recently been ill, it is customary to say that he is pale around the gills. As age creeps on us, it always shows its mark by the emaciation and the flabby appearance of the neck. A shapely neck is an even finer example of virile manhood than are good hips. Of the two it is more apt to attract your first glance. All animals, the horse, lion or tiger, manifest their superb carriage in their proudly arched necks. It is just the same with man. If he holds his head straight with his shoulders back, and walks with a lilt to his stride and a spring to his step, he owns a real neck. It is one part of your body you cannot successfully cover. Everywhere you look you will always find more scrawny necks, protruding Adam's apples, or hollowed necks, than you will find straight columnar necks of the vibrant man.

The most important muscles that surround the neck are the sterno mastoid and the trapezius, and the seven vertebrae that support the head are known as the cervical spines. The most characteristic feature of the neck is the shortness of the cervical spines. This gives to the neck the distinct advantage of being able to bend backwards to an acute angle, without any of the attendant dangers that are liable to appear in a lower back bend. If this was not the case, wrestlers would never be able to stand the grueling to which the head locks subject them. The natural formation of the sterno-mastoid also helps to make this possible. It is the prominent muscle projecting on the side of the neck that separates the anterior from the posterior triangle, fitting obliquely in the neck. In other words, it forms a triangle from the back of the head to the front of the throat. Actually it is fastened to the occipital bone behind the ear and to the sternum bone. Because of the position of this pair of muscles they give the head a triple movement. Acting alone, either muscle singly, turns the head to either side. Working together they hold the head forward. They also act as extraordinary muscles of inspiration, by raising the sternum and clavicles in a movement similar to raising the face upwards.

Just for a moment, I am going to digress by asking you to call to mind the neck condition of the lower animals. Did you ever notice how much larger their neck is in proportion to their bodies than is that of a man. Just try to hold the head of a collie dog, and see what a time you will have. Ten to one he will break away. A larger dog would haul you all over. Just so the necks of a dog, bear, or gorilla are more powerful than of a horse or a cow. The necks of the latter have not the fullness that the others have, and by twisting their heads they can be thrown and held down, providing the pressure is applied to the side of the head and neck. The horse and the cow, like the deer, stag or moose, apply their strength in other directions, such as tossing and pulling. Some breeds of cows and horses have shorter and, therefore, more powerful necks, just the same as the difference between long-necked and short-necked men. However, this is not what I started out to tell you. The real issue I wanted to discuss goes back to evolution. It is the result of something we have lost in our march to civilization and which has been retained in the lower animal. If you make a close study of the sterno-mastoid, you will find that on either side these fleshy columns are separated from each other by a fibrous partition. This is a feeble relic in man of the stout elastic ligament which is so often met with among the lower animals. Our erect posture caused it to degenerate, but in the animal that walks on all fours it has to be very strong to support the head in the horizontal position.

I mention this fact because I think it may interest you and because I have been questioned along these lines. Although we have no intention of walking on all fours again, yet any muscular action seen in other living creatures, and not common to man, is always interesting to me.

The next muscle of importance is the Trapezius. Although mainly a back muscle, yet it is finally attached to the occipital bone forming the major part of the breadth of the back of the neck. This muscle operates from different positions, but ordinarily it is never so powerful at the back of the neck as it is in the back itself. A defect in this muscle always shows itself in the scooped hollow so often prominent on the back of the neck. Now of these two particular pairs of muscles, the sterno-mastoid is the more frequently employed. There is hardly any daily cause for vigorous play of the trapezius, unless someone places his hands playfully upon the top of your head and pulls it down. Then in order to resist, you will have to pull backwards and this brings the trapezius into action. However, I find that they develop quite rapidly; more rapidly than the sterno-mastoid.

In other chapters you may have noticed how often I have referred to the way in which vigorous muscle stimulation was caused by nerve vibration. The very life, and the volatile power of your muscles depend upon the

163

nerve supply contained in each. The power of the generative supply of the nervous system is largely dependent upon the condition of the neck. It is here that we find the source of our nervous activity. It continues all down the spine, from which it shoots out its branches to stimulate the whole body. Every man who is endowed with a powerful neck is possessed of great concentrated energy. This rule never fails. Look at any athlete who is vigorously strong and you will see that the tape measure gives him a much larger neck than the average. It is a fixed fact in the minds of everybody that a strong body must have a strong neck. Sculptors and artists never overlook this point, although I doubt whether all of them realize the true importance of the neck, and the part it plays in our health, and how it decides for us how much concentrated strength we each have.

One time when I was up in the highlands of Canada, around Golden Lake, I noticed a beautiful body of water flowing through the hills. It branched into many little streams, spreading its fertility wherever the streams traversed, just as the nerves fertilize the body, stimulating growth, and establishing a better order of physical life.

To allow such unsightly things as a hollow neck, pocket holes, or a billiard ball Adam's apple to exist is not being fair to yourself. By just applying yourself to a few well selected exercises these faults can be overcome. The one form of exercise to which the neck will not respond is free movements. You must remember that the neck is very powerfully constructed and when fairly developed carries a great mass of muscle about it in comparison to its length. Yet you do not have to jump into a lot of vigorous exercises all at once. Take it easy, and coax your neck, rather than force it. Some commence by using the hands as a form of resistance. If your neck is very weak, it is not a bad idea to practice that for a couple of weeks. But if you want to test your neck strength, you will find that it can easily resist any pressure from the hands. In other words, the neck is stronger than the arms. Therefore, it is not logical to expect to achieve any distinct success by employing a weaker resistance. The wrestler's bridge is a favorite exercise with most body builders, but they have the wrong idea of this exercise. Seemingly, it is thought that wrestlers develop their powerful neck from bridging. True, from bridging, but not in bridging. What I mean is that their development is obtained from going up into the bridge and not in holding the bridge. Body builders generally assume the wrestler's bridge and then push a bar-bell to arms' length several times while in that position. It becomes merely an arm exercise in a support. I consider a bridge nothing else but a support. No man can lift anything like the weight he can support in the wrestler's bridge. The

spines in the neck merely act as a prop, as the head is actually forced between the shoulders.

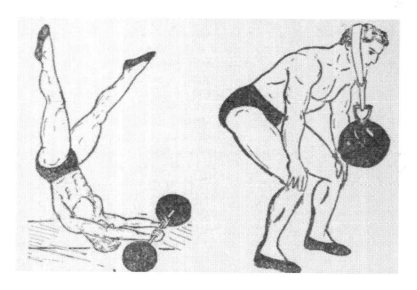

Some find the bridge very difficult to form. There is nothing to it. What happens is this. The exerciser will lie on the floor with his feet drawn up towards the buttocks; then he will try to pry himself up, and find that he cannot. The reason for this is that he has not considered certain points, and the distance between his head and heels is too great, and he is unable to make the grade to the crown of his head. What he should do is to first draw the heels as close to the body as possible, then place the hands behind the head, and draw the head well under towards the shoulders. This done, thrust with the legs so that the body weight is forced towards the head.

Now the best way to obtain the right effect upon the neck muscles is to bend the neck at the shoulders when in the wrestler's bridge position, and simply lower the shoulders to the ground. Then by prying and pressing the head against the floor, raise into the bridge again. Full action is obtained from the neck muscles this way. Some make the mistake of swaying the body up on to the head. That is wrong. Let your neck do the work, and you will find the exercise considerably more vigorous. When you feel you have become too strong for this movement, just hold a light barbell at arms' length throughout the exercise, and you will get just the right kind of resistance to continue your progression.

This exercise will get the trapezius muscles nicely, but if you want to bring the sterno-mastoids into play all you have to do is twist the head from side to side, while in the bridge position, so that each time you bridge you roll onto the temple. However, be sure and make it a neck movement and not a motion done with the sway of the body. The further you twist to the side of the face the better will these neck columns work.

A man who has a good chest, and broad shoulders, will generally find it less difficult to develop a sturdy neck. Some people have a long, slim neck that seems to cause the shoulders to slope. Invariably, we find that the man with the long, slim neck has short clavicles, which makes his neck look worse than it is. Of course, we cannot stretch the clavicles. The only thing left to do is to concentrate upon widening the shoulders and building up the deltoids. Wide shoulders and a deep chest allow greater space for the neck muscles to spread. Then, on the other hand, they require a larger-sized neck to look like anything.

By way of variation, here are a few more exercises that you may like better, and which I can guarantee will give you the best results, although it is wise to practice them all. You commence by making a sling, with a hook attached, which will fit on the head and fasten below the chin. Take up your position with the hands upon the knees and the body bent well forwards from the waist. Then hook a kettle-bell to the sling and exercise the neck by bending the head forward so that the chin touches the chest. From that angle raise the head backward as far as possible. For the next exercise, turn the head from side to side. The first will get the trapezius, and the second exercise will catch the sterno-mastoids. Another good exercise is performed by lying on the back on a couch, with the head and neck protruding past the end. Allow the sling to rest upon the forehead with the kettle-bell hanging under the head. Now lower the head backward towards the floor as far as you can, without having the sling slip off the fore-, head. Then concentrate strongly and raise the head by bringing the chin towards the chest.

If you want a really vigorous exercise, you will find the following movement sufficient for your needs. It is a great favorite of mine. In the first place, you should secure a good cushion or pillow for this exercise and the same should be used when bridging.

Load a barbell pretty heavily, and place it at the back of the head. Throw your hands over and grasp the bar and see that the cushion is placed under the head. You will be lying full length upon the floor. Now draw your legs up quickly, pulling the knees to the chest, and like lightning shoot the legs upwards, and at the same time pry with the neck muscles and pull on the bar. If you do this properly you will be standing on your head at the conclusion of the movement, with your hands holding to the bar for support and to steady your balance. As you lower yourself back to the original position, just bend the neck and roll down onto the shoulders and back. This can be done slowly if you pull sufficiently on the bar, with fine results. As you become more proficient at this exercise you can even go up slowly. I often do this when in bed, using the bed rail in place of the barbell. This exercise helped to make my neck so strong that I was able to perform the following stunt, which I have rarely seen duplicated. When it was duplicated, only a man who had a very powerful neck did the feat. It goes something like this. I sit on the floor with arms folded, then quickly roll backwards, and as the head touches the floor, I press vigorously and thrust my legs upwards. The force, or throw of the neck, is so great that my body- weight is thrown into the air and I land on my feet in the same manner as though I had performed a back somersault. It is a very spectacular stunt, and one which I used to include in my exhibitions with great success.

I used to get a great workout with a little practice I included always in my wrestling training. I have advocated it a lot to many neck builders, who find difficulty in making the neck grow. The replies have all been very enthusiastic and I believe you will enjoy it. You need a partner, which may be a slight drawback, but one I believe you can easily overcome. Allow your friend to take a front head lock on you. To do this you both stand facing each other. You bend forward, and your partner wraps his right arm around your head, locking his hands to increase the resistance. Now do not get the idea in your head that all you have to do is break away. Nothing like that. Instead, pull, push and twist, hauling your partner all over with the movements. You will get such neck power that with very little training it will enable you to swing your partner off his feet. It has an exhilarating effect upon the spine. You can actually feel your nervous vitality increase. Wrestlers always have good necks. This is the reason they last so long in athletics. No matter how severe the neck play, there is never any danger of blood congestion, as some try to make believe. If there was such a danger wrestlers would be the first to show the effects. As a matter of fact, wrestlers can rest while in the bridge formation. I have seen wrestlers, when in the bridge formation, picked up and crashed down time after time, but with no results. Standing on their heads in crotch holds they are capable of head spinning and resisting all their opponent's downward pressure.

For a boxer to resist a knockout punch the stronger the neck is formed the better off he will be. In the less-cultured days of the boxing ring less clever boxers made a practice of catching blows on the side of the head. Such boxers always displayed a strong neck. These are extreme examples, but they go to show the extreme limits to which the neck muscles are capable of resisting without any detrimental effects.

In many of the European coast fishing towns the fisher people use their heads for carrying their baskets of fish, as coal heavers carry coal on their backs. The finest examples are found among the Bretons of France, and among the people of the east coast of England. I remember on first seeing these people how impressed I was with the fine carriage of the women. I was later amazed to see these same women balancing on their heads a basket loaded with fish, and walking along as though the load was nothing. They had beautifully shaped necks, which were undoubtedly the reason for the wonderful development of their bodies. Short skirts, with bare feet, and very short sleeves in their shirt waists, with the throat, shoulders and bosom partly exposed, made up their costume. Never since have I seen such magnificent specimens of womanhood. In my mind they stand out as the finest members of the other sex that can be found.

Neck strength is a wonderful asset. It is always evinced by a beautiful shapeliness that never fails to please the eye. It is something to strive for and to be proud to own. Exercise will make such a possession easily attainable. All the greatest men I have ever known, who displayed great concentrated energy, carried a columnar neck and a perfect bodily poise. George Hackenschmidt had one of the most imposing necks I ever saw. Every part was perfectly molded. Nordquest, Travis, Steinborn, Cadine, Dandurand, Fournier, Klein and Coulter, among a few that I can immediately call to mind, all own beautifully formed necks, which are pillars of power, and their wonderful general physique and remarkable strength is positive proof of how a columnar neck can invigorate the whole body with its creative nerve force.

CHAPTER XII
STRENGTHENING THE WEAKEST LINK IN THE SPINAL CHAIN

When I was a little chap and things were not going just the way they should, my dad would say to me by way of encouragement, "Put your back to the wheel, sonny, and you'll pull through." It helped to put the sand in me, and I'd come back just that ,much stronger. However, as I grew to manhood and left the shelter of the parental wing, I found the necessity of putting my back to the wheel greater than ever, to meet the obligations of manhood.

It has become habitual with mankind to use certain expressions until they have a world of meaning, and while it is understood that the little saying of my dad, and millions of others, is just one that can be applied in many senses, yet it holds a lesson. It tells the mind in more ways than one, that the back is the source of our man power. "You are just as old as your back," the family physician will tell you, and he is right. Without a strong back you can't get anywhere. A weak back weakens all of your natural resources, and you become a living wreck.

If I asked ten men on the street to place their finger on what they considered to be the weakest part of the spine, nine would instinctively name the small of the back. The tenth one might hesitate, but understanding would overcome that hesitancy and he would side in with the other nine. That is where all the back aches and pains that seem to sap the life and energy of a man originate. But why put up with it? There is a cause for this unnatural condition, and a natural way to overcome that cause.

The lumbar region, and sacrovertebral sector of the spine, are the parts of the back that are prone to weakness. Like weakness in any other part of the body, this is all due to lack of muscular toning, but other parts of the body can lack proper muscular toning, and yet never have the injurious effect upon our general health that a muscular weakness in the small of the back has. The main reason is that other muscles do not envelop the important organs of life, which are found in the sector formed by the spine from the base of the last rib down to the sacrum. Of course, the heart and lungs are extremely important, but look at the protective agencies that surround them. The bony structure of the ribs, and a mass of muscle back and front, that are not as prone to deterioration as is the case with the muscles of the lumbar region. Where you find a weak back, you find a weak abdomen, and with the degeneration of muscular tissue in the back and abdomen, what have you to protect the organs of assimilation and evacuation? There are no other structural supports to help this part of the spine, which exists alone in its bending, twisting and moving with the thousand and one daily actions of the body.

No matter what part of the muscular body you may have under cultivation, a fact that you should always bear in mind is that wherever the muscular organism is low, the nerve generation is low too. You know then what the results must be. Low vitality and virility.

The vertebral column consists of thirty-three segments or vertebrae, which are divided into five sections and named according to the regions through which they pass. I think, while we are on the subject, I might as well name these parts as a source of information for future reference. Now all these five sectors of the thirty- three vertebrae are divided into two other classes, and are known as the movable, or true spine, and the fixed, or false spine. The first seven are known as the cervical and cover the space from the head to the shoulders. The next twelve are the thoracic, that cover the costal, or rib region. Next five are the lumbar. Next five the sacral, the remaining four are known as the coccygeal. Our interest is centered upon the lumbar and sacral sector, but more particularly the lumbar region. So let us begin by concentrating upon these five segments.

Due to the fact that these five vertebrae stand alone, they are quite a bit heavier than the other movable vertebrae, and are supported and controlled by the muscles which surround them. Now if you carefully study the spinal column, you will see that it has an interrupted connection. That is, between each vertebrae there exists a space. This space is filled up by a cartillagus pad, or cushion, and from each vertebra there runs a nerve which branches from the sciatic nerve. With each nerve runs a feeder. These nerves stimulate the muscles in their activity according to the degree of their health. Often these nerves become impinged or affected, and in most cases the nerve injury is the result of the poor condition of the muscles in the lumbar region. These happenings are quite commonplace. Perhaps you have been bent over in a stooped position longer than you were accustomed to. Maybe you stopped to pick up something and you got a kink in your back. The object does not necessarily have to be heavy to cause this. Then again, you might have been reaching too high, or it may have been a cold that lodged in the small of the back, or the kidneys were out of order. In the first three conditions, a vertebral displacement has probably occurred; in the last two the blood circulation has not been up to the mark, and its sluggish condition has allowed some affection to invade this part. Of course, there can be, and undoubtedly are, other causes of these conditions, but I am sure these muscular conditions are a very prominent factor in causing all the trouble.

It goes without saying that if the muscles of the back are up to par the blood condition will also be good, and when the latter condition is good the nervous system is healthy.

Anyhow, let us take a little look at the back in the lumbar region. We don't need a skeleton; we will consider the average person in the nude. In the first place you will see that right above the hips the back arches in a forward curve. If the muscles are well developed, you will see a groove, with long, fleshy columns flanking each side of the spine. If these fleshy columns were not there then you will see the backbone sticking out in a pronounced ridge. Now there is such a thing as having too deep a spinal depression. It is a condition of curvature, and I believe such a spine is much weaker than most other spinal conditions. These backs are always weak when it comes to holding or pushing any objects overhead, or doing any work that calls for overhead action, or carrying heavy objects in the arms with the weight across the chest. You see the movable vertebrae have a downward inclination. That is, they are meant to support a weight in the perpendicular, but if the arch is too pronounced the pressure is not entirely perpendicular, and a vertebral displacement or compression is more readily affected. By developing the spinal erectus muscles this condition can be improved. Now the prominent backbone, which generally brings about the lazy humpback condition, is caused through lack of muscular quantity, and the possessors of such backs cannot stand lifting any objects off the ground. Most backs have this defect and most people cannot stand an hour shoveling coal in the cellar or snow off the pavement. They get a lame back of some kind. The muscle is not there, and all the strain is thrown upon the spine. A nervous reaction and irritation is always being caused, which generally develops into lumbago and kindred troubles. When the nerves are affected the muscles do not receive their natural flow of energy and they become stagnant.

What most often happens is this. Nerve irritation burns up a lot of energy, which breaks down a certain amount of tissues, and due to the fact that the muscles are not as active as they should be, a carbonic substance accumulates. Not only does this substance clog the muscle cells, but it accumulates around the vertebral segment. In time this substance forms a scale, which in process of accumulation becomes lodged between the movable segments. Then an impingement is created against the nerve or nerve feeder, which is dangerous in either case. From this source originates the curse of the backache. Wherever there is a lack of muscle something has to help out, and the nerves work overtime trying to charge the muscles with the necessary electricity to secure the action. It works out much the same way as starting the motor in an automobile when the spark plugs are fouled. The batteries work overtime to supply the necessary ignition.

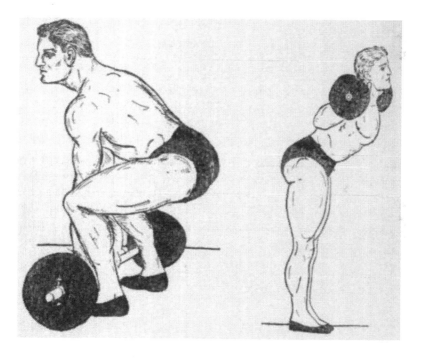

Faulty positions have a lot to do with our back troubles. For instance, when a man leans over to pick up an object he does so with a round back. Wherever a round back is employed the muscles of the small of the back flatten out instead of contracting. Now the vertebrae in the spine open fanwise, producing a wide space between each segment. The lumbar section is no different, and whenever you lift with a round back with flattened muscles, you are in the position that most readily causes the vertebrae to become displaced. The muscles, instead of being contracted, are extended. No support is there to reinforce the spine, and the vertebrae, in trying their best to work alone, slip out of line, a condition which may call for a chiropractic adjustment. When the back is flattened, just notice the difference. Why; the erector spinae muscles bulge like pillars of steel as they contract to fulfill their duty, which their name explains— "erect the spine." This is as it should be. Also, instead of a vertebral separation, the vertebrae close together into one apparently solid column, which positively prevents any such thing as a vertebral displacement.

A few years ago an exercise was taught, and widely used, in which the exerciser stood on a stool while holding a weight in both hands. Then the exerciser was supposed to bend forward, stiff-kneed, and see how far past the toes he could allow his hands to travel, and from that position raise himself erect. That is one of the worst exercises any one can do* How can your erector spinae muscles erect the spine when they are not contracted? It is not. logical, apart from the unnatural position into which it throws the vertebrae. Go to a chiropractor and learn what he will tell you. He will say, "Exercise, but do not practice touching the toes." I asked one chiropractor friend why he advised that omission, and he frankly told me that it always had a tendency to undo what he had corrected. He knew the effect on the spine all right, but he was not a student of anatomy and did not know the muscular action. When I explained the muscular action to him he understood clearly how right he was. Lifting with a rounded back also has a bad effect on the abdomen, as it causes a great compression. I make all my pupils use a flat back, which apart from correcting any faulty spinal position, does not bring about the compression of the abdomen. In the lift known as the two hands Dead Lift, and Hands Alone, I immediately caution a lifter when I see his back begin to round.

The erector spinae muscles are very important. They are also very peculiar muscles, due to the manner in which they branch out. Their proper name is the sacrospinal, because they originate in the region of the sacrum and run all the way up the spine to the skull. The muscles of the back are arranged in four series according to their attachments, and their order is as follows: Vertebro-scapular, vertebro humeral, vertebro cranial and vertebral. Of this group the erector spinae are the vertebro cranial, and vertebro costal, because they are attached to the cranium or skull, and the ribs. They commence at the dorsum of the sacrum and follow up the spines of the sacral and lumbar regions. It really is a deep muscle, practically covered by the fascia or membranus attachments of the latissimus dorsi muscles. They bulge very heavily in the lumbar region, where they are most prominent, and taper away under the latissimus dorsi and trapezius muscles. One on each side of the backbone, they form additional spinal columns that can be developed into really massive pillars of muscle. I have seen some athletes with such heavy development here that the mass was almost the depth of my fingers. Get these muscles built up right, and there will be little to fear from lumbago or any of its kindred back disorders.

The latissimus dorsi muscle is the big muscle that covers all the small of the back. It is known as a vertebro humeral, because its origination is on the spine and it becomes attached in the bicepital groove of the humerus bone.

Weight lifters, shot putters, hammer throwers, and scullers, all have powerfully developed backs. This is especially true of weight lifters and scullers. A favorite pastime with scullers is pulling the stick. The contestants sit on the floor and place the soles of their feet against each other. Then they take a stick and both take hold. The object is for the stronger man to pull the other off the floor. Of course, this is a sculler's specialty, and if he is not good at this stunt, he is not good at sculling, just as a lifter unable to raise an one hundred pound bag of flour overhead with one hand would not be good at lifting. However, the best man I ever saw at pulling the stick weighed one hundred and forty-five pounds, and had never sat in a shell in his life. He was a great track star, with a distinguished athletic record while in the army, but he is otherwise unknown. Arthur Latcham was his name. He and I chummed together and I have seen him pull large, powerful men with ease. Honestly, I would like to see the man who could pull him. He stuck me more than once. He was an enthusiastic bar bell man and it was from this source he obtained his power. He had a great fondness for that pastime. There is an interesting stunt which is similar and practiced a lot by lumberjacks. They pit their strength against horses instead of men, by hitching a horse to a whiffle-tree with the tugs passing on each side of a tree. The lumberjack takes up his position with the whiffletree held in the bend of his elbows and his feet firmly planted against the trunk of the tree. The object is to resist the horse's pull a few seconds. Some men have resisted the pull of a team of horses. This feat calls for all-round bodily strength, but the moment the back bends it is all over.

Exercises for the erector spinae muscles are quite numerous. Two that I know you will find interesting and productive of good results follow. Place a bar bell, about forty pounds in weight, across the shoulders. Allow the feet to be spaced from twelve to eighteen inches apart and keep the knees locked. Take hold of the bar with each hand and begin to bend forward until the body is at right angles with the waist, and then return to the erect position. However, always keep the back flat and straight.

While the bar bell is held in the same position, bend sideways from the hips—bending from the hips allows the body to lean at a more acute angle—moving from side to side. The erector spinae muscles will show up very prominently in these movements. When I want to get a good view of these powerful back erectors I generally ask the exerciser to clasp his hands at the back of the head, and then bend over backwards and sideways. Take for instance Sam Kramer, Massimo, Steinborn, and among the lighter men, Fournier and Klein. When any of these men strike that position the erector spinae muscles have the appearance of huge twisted cables. Any movement that twists the body or bends it brings these muscles into action.

The latissimi dorsi are muscles which are entirely surfacial, covering the erector spinae muscles, spreading across the small of the back, slightly covering part of the serratus magnus in their process of insertion upon the humerus bone. They are very powerful, and, as their name implies, they are the broadest of the back muscles. While they have a lot to do with the small of the back, they have a lot to do with broadening the upper back. Movements that pull a weight to the chest from the ground, and that thrust the weight overhead with either one or two arms, are good developers for these muscles. But of the two series of muscles, the sacrospinalis are the more directly important to the spine. They are known as the muscles of posture and, as I said before, they originate down in the sacrum region and cover the area of the fixed or immovable spines, as well as of the lumbar section. If these muscles do not receive any active stimulation, they seem to deteriorate quickly and lose energy. They lose their power of contraction and their elasticity and the living cells of the muscles become clogged. Then the spine is affected in a more dangerous manner. The hardest ache or pain to get rid of is one in the region of the sacrum of the spine.

A peculiarity of the spine is that when we rest at night we grow taller. During the daytime the direct pressure of our body upon the vertebrae causes the cartillegus pads to flatten somewhat, but in our nightly process of recuperation they elongate. It is with the idea of causing a greater elongation of these pads that the people work, who claim they can increase their height. In my estimation it is a foolish and a dangerous practice. These pads are not muscles. If you are meant to be tall you will be tall, and if short you will be short. Exercise will stimulate the growth of the spine and get out of it all that nature intended, but you must work through the muscles. The bar bell man gets the most out of all things that are muscular, his muscles become supple, strong and active. Make the small of your back the dynamo of your spine and help yourself by putting steel in it from proper intensive training.

CHAPTER XIII
CREATING INTENSE VITALITY BY ABDOMINAL DEVELOPMENT

After explaining the conditions that control the small of the back, I will now draw your attention to the same region, but to the front of the torso, which we might safely term the pit of the body. Just as the condition of the small of the back controls vitality, so does the condition of the abdomen control the vital sources of digestion. It is what the organs of digestion get from the foods that really supplies the whole body with its energy. In the chapter on Curative Exercise I explained how the various particles of food were transferred into the blood stream, and conveyed to the various sources, to become finally absorbed by the living cells of the tissues. You are fully aware of the fact that if the muscular wall that protects the abdomen is not taken care of, many conditions will arise that will be detrimental to the lasting life of your organs. The one great object in our life, as body builders, is to increase the resistance of the muscles, internal and external, against the ravages of time and disease. We know that to do this we must build the muscles of the body to the highest state of their physical perfection. Fine arms, legs, neck and back arc great, but without the fully developed torso they are all obtained in vain. The old saw still says you are just as strong as your weakest link, and it is only too true.

I wonder if you have noticed one thing missing in all of the chapters I have written in this volume, particularly where I have discussed building up the various muscles of the body. I think you have, but to make this positive in your mind I will allude to it. With the exception of the chapter on finger strength, I have not mentioned any great feats of strength, or made any comparison of how much this man did, or that man did, to show the possibilities of the muscles outlined for cultivation. This may be considered strange, but I have a definite object in mind. Just this. I have known many aspirants for better bodies to become totally discouraged by such comparisons. Others defeat their purpose by believing they should come pretty close to what the best have done.

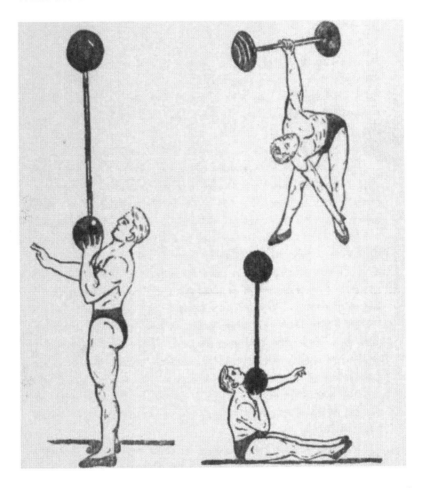

You should remember that the fine achievements of those great exponents of muscle culture were the result of intensive training over a period of time. By following the same example as they, you also can succeed. Therefore, it is my earnest desire to teach the reader the principles rather than demonstrate the results of body-building. The latter will inevitably follow. I know you are interested in all those things, but I have taken care of them in other chapters. What I am concerned with now is building you over, and the abdomen is a good place to impress you with the fact, with the reminder that the condition of your abdomen is going to decide many things for you. If you have a strongly built abdomen you will have a strong back; but, that does not mean if you have a strong back you have a strong abdomen. Oh, no! Many men who have allowed themselves to slip still retain a strong back, but the obesity of the abdomen tells another story. Yet, we can always associate a well-formed torso with a well-formed back.

The muscles of the abdomen consist of the four twin sections, that armor-like, form a muscular wall of protection for the contents of the abdomen and are aided by the muscles of the sides, which we term the external oblique muscles. The abdominals are fastened to the breast-bone and to the pelvis, with the external oblique muscles running obliquely through the groin to their insertion. These muscles help to erect the body in all forward and side movements, but display their great power of construction in bending movements. They are very flexible, and can be actually controlled better than any other group of muscles. Unfortunately, they seem to be the first muscles in the body that are prone to degenerate more rapidly than the erector spinae muscle in the sacrum region, or the muscles of the neck. They lose their elasticity and contractile power, which is proven by the enormous percentage of obese stomachs, sagging abdomens and the constant liability to hernia.

You have noticed the formation of these muscles on the abdomen, ridges of fleshy cables that run horizontally across the body. In the well formed body builder this is termed the "wash board." They give that appearance when

183

they are contracted, four ridges rolling upon each other. The last section commences on the line of the naval, and has a long conical construction tapering away in the pelvis. None of these muscles are distinctly separated from each other. Acting more like sympathetic muscles, they are attached to each other by a thin membranous fascia. The most popular exercise is the "sit up." The exerciser lies on the floor with a light weight held behind the neck, and has some heavy object over his feet to hold him down, as he performs the exercise. This may be a bar-bell, or else the feet are placed under the edge of a bureau. Pulling on the bar at the back of the neck the exerciser rises into the "sit up" position. Common as is this exercise, many have a lot of trouble with it, and no wonder, because they keep the back too straight. The back should be rounded as much as possible so that the distance between the face and the knees is shortened. It is in this rounded position that the abdominals obtain their strongest contraction and benefit. My advice to those who find it so difficult is to commence the exercise from the sit-up position, rather than from lying down. The back can be better rounded at the start, and the exerciser should lower his body to the floor in a rolling movement. Just as soon as he feels the broad of the back touch the floor, he should immediately begin to rise again. Only a very light weight is required to start. Professional athletes used to use the

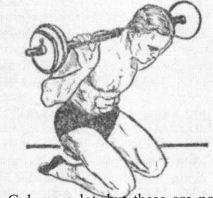

Roman Chair and Roman Column a lot, but these are not very handy in a bedroom, so we might as well forget them, apart from the fact that they are also difficult to purchase.

However, by allowing the small of the back to rest across the seat of a chair, with the feet placed under some object, the exerciser can get some good abdominal action by pulling a weight over the face and rising to a "sit up" position on the chair, a pair of dumb bells are handier in this position than a bar bell.

Yet another exercise that is good is to kneel on the floor with the knees wide apart and a light bar-bell held across the back of the neck. By bending forward as low as possible, with a rounded back, you will find it not as easy to straighten the body back to the erect position.

Another form of developing the abdominal muscles has been widely practiced of late years, but it is not so successful for many reasons. As a method of muscle building it is not very important, but as a means of massaging, and stimulating the digestive tracts, it is good. Better known as "muscle control," it was first written of in America by Ottley R. Coulter, who was a great exponent of this method, besides being a pupil of the famous Maxick, who introduced the study in England. Maxick could perform some remarkable controls, and for a while this method of training became the rage. A few of the controls are the complete isolation of the diaphragm, the double isolation of the rectus abdominals—which is better known as the "rope," because it creates the impression that the athlete had swallowed a piece of heavy rope, and it was standing upright in the cavity of the abdomen. Another is the single abdominal isolation. In this last feat, just one side of the abdominals are tensed, and the other side shows only a deep hollow cavity. In the full isolation of the diaphragm, the stomach and all the intestinal organs seem to disappear, leaving a huge hollow. Both fists can be buried in the large hole formed under the thorax. What really happens is that by taking a few deep intakes of breath, and exhaling same, a vacuum is created that sucks or draws in the abdominal space. The same happens in all of the abdominal controls, the only difference being that a different muscular control is called into existence operating with the created vacuum. An athlete does not necessarily have to possess any remarkable development to be able to perform these controls, although the better abdominal development the more effective are the controls displayed. I would much rather see a body culturist concentrate on building up the muscles of his abdomen rather than put the same amount of time in learning these controls. Take the abdominal development of Siegmund Klein, or Ottley Coulter. There is something very impressive in the ridges of muscle that ripple over either of their abdomens. It is far more worthwhile to secure these results first. The controls will come easily afterwards. I have seen Mr. Coulter display even Pauperts ligaments in some of his controls. To my mind that is the only demonstration I ever saw of these ligaments.

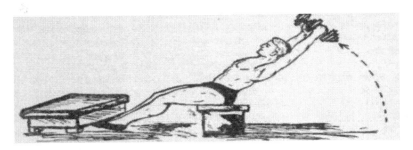

In the chapter on Curative Exercises I gave a number of exercises, and among them was the "sit up," which I did not explain as fully there as here, as stated at that time. For muscle building it is all right and has a great influence in decreasing the stomach. For the muscles on the lower abdomen the leg-raising exercise is the best. Next, attention should be given to the external oblique muscles, which fit on the side of the body from beneath the ribs, and are flanked on the back by the latissimus dorsi. They run into the groin, and help to make the superb development seen on the torso of Klein and Coulter. If you ever pay attention to the Grecian torsos, and other statues, you will quickly notice the crest of muscle that seems to bulge over the side of the hip bone. That is the muscle. Grecian torsos did not die with the decline of that Empire. They are one of nature's possessions that the efforts of man can always hold. There are just as finely built men today as two thousand years ago, and the columns of the various physical culture magazines constantly display them.

Raising a weight to arms' length, while bending over sideways, is an important exercise for the external oblique muscle. So is holding a weight at arms' length overhead and bending over sideways so that you are able to touch the toes with the other hand. The one thing you have to watch in this exercise is to keep the lifting leg straight throughout the exercise. A little feat that is very attractive and helps considerably to build up these muscles is done as follows: Raise a bar bell to arms' length overhead with one hand, and while keeping it at arms' length, lie flat on the back on the floor. Still keeping it at arms' length, rise to the erect position. In fact, this stunt stimulates into action all the muscles in the abdominal region, but due to all the side bending necessitated, the external obliques receive a little extra play.

Balance a bar bell on the hand, and as you continue to balance it thus you will be obliged to juggle it in order to maintain the balance. All the movement caused by the juggling will be controlled by the muscles in the waist region. When you get good at it, you can make a deep knee bend, and then sit on the floor still balancing the bar bell, and rise to the erect position. You really will be surprised to see just how much play is given to the abdomen and side muscles by this little feat. It is necessary that the boxer should have a well-muscled abdomen, otherwise the solar plexus blow will soon put him out of commission. It appears that there is a little knot of nerves at the pit of the stomach that are very sensitive, and a well-placed blow there seems to paralyze the nervous system temporarily. Some boxers are very proud of their abdominal strength, and I have seen them stand up and allow others to punch them all over the abdomen as hard as they like. On one occasion I saw a man strike an old pugilist with a ten-pound dumb-bell, but so well formed were his muscles that they absorbed the blow without his flinching. It is not an uncommon feat to see some men allow others to jump on their stomach, even from the height of a table, and with no ill effects. Frank Dennis, allowed an automobile to run over his stomach while flat upon his back on the ground, with no protection.

Personally, I do not approve of such stunts. They are not necessary, but still they go to prove to what a remarkable extent the abdomen can be developed, and the terrific resistance of which the abdominal muscles are capable.

CHAPTER XIV
BANISHING ROUND SHOULDERS AND PROTRUDING SHOULDER BLADES

"Straighten up there. Haven't you any backbone in you?" Did you ever hear a top sergeant yell this at some raw rookie? I will bet you did if you were ever in the army. There is more talk of this kind than anything else where the army is breaking in its new men. However, we do not have to go to any army training quarters to see such specimens, for they are as thick upon the streets as hair on a dog. Humpbacks, round shoulders, or shoulder blades that stick out like razor blades are a common sight. It really is a shame when you think of it, and realize how the internal organs of the thorax become congested through such negligence. I have often thought that the characteristics which are developed between the age of fifteen and eighteen are those that will control the young man's future, both mentally and physically. Around that age, we see more slouchy boys than well set-up young chaps. To walk erect at sixteen years of age generally brings contemptuous comments from others of the same age, who tell the rest of the "gang" that that guy likes to show off, or thinks he is somebody. Well, it is the age of the growing boy, who wants to be a man before his time. The boy, some mock, is invariably their pride on the diamond, or the gridiron, and more or less all the boys admire him, but they feel they want to be just a bit different. It is right here that their mistake is made. The gawky boy effects a slouchy walk, which makes his shoulder blades stick out and spoils the natural carriage of his back. Then, when he begins to straighten up, he finds the new position a little distressing. But, I will say this, that if there is one part of the body on which the effect of exercise is felt almost immediately, it is the back. Just for an example, take a bar bell loaded to about fifty or seventy-five pounds, and press it to arms' length overhead a few times. Then place it on the floor and stand up and walk. If you raised the weight two or three extra times by just determining you were going to lift that bar bell as many times as you could, you will feel a very forcible back- pull, as you walk. For a few steps the unusually erect carriage will make your stride feel different. Anyhow, you will notice how much more erect you were after the exercise than before. Of course, this will not be permanent, but it will only take a few weeks of intensive bar bell training to make the result permanent.

You see it is like this, from, lack of proper use, the muscles on the broad of the back lose their natural power of contraction. They become stringy and weak. The result is that the scapula bones, or shoulder blades, are not held in place, and the arms seem to become too heavy for the shoulders.

Some time, when you are attending a swimming pool, just look the boys over and see if you do not find these conditions. First take a really ordinary person, and on the upper body you will notice that there appears to be no trace of the existence of the latissimus dorsi muscles, the serratus magnus, deltoids, trapezius and arm triceps. At the best, they will only appear in a rudimentary condition. Is there any wonder they have such unnatural upper body development? Turn your attention to the earnest exercise fan, and you see a completely different type of manhood.

The serratus magnus has a scapular origin, and if it only exists in a mediocre condition, how can one expect the shoulder blades to be in their original place? The trapezius is the muscle that covers the most of the shoulder blade. It is a large triangular slab of muscle that is attached to the spine covering both the cervical and the thoracic part of the spine, or, as we would commonly say, from the base of the skull down to the small of the back. It slants from the lumbar region up to the shoulder girdle, and then travels along the clavicle, or collar-bone. This is what gives this muscle its threefold origin. Even with this, I used to wonder why it contracted so strangely. If you clasp your hands behind the back and press downwards, bringing the shoulder blades together, you will notice right at the base of the neck a bunch of muscle, shaped like a crater. It has a hollow depression, but if you pull on your head with your hands you see the trapezius forms into a cable of muscle, something like a continuation of the erector spinae muscles. I found out why it functioned this way. From the lumbar region the muscular fibers slant up toward the girdle of the shoulders, and from there they go in the opposite direction, slanting from the site of the collar-bone to the base of the skull. This is the reason why greater neck power can be employed by lifting the head in a spiral movement than in a straight, backward movement. With this knowledge of the trapezius, I acquired more respect for them, although I used to think, like the majority of exercise fans, that the latissimus dorsi was the most important muscle in the broad of the back. Hand balancers, and ground tumblers, always have a finely developed upper back, as have wrestlers, but unquestionably bar bell fans and weight lifters build up the most powerful backs.

I once owned a real old book on physical education. In those \ days the anatomical names were not so well understood as they are now. I remember that the trapezius was spoken of as the "monk's cowl" muscle. I can quite well understand why it was termed that, as it takes the appearance of the cowl of a monk as it spreads along the collar-bone. I have heard some real old-timers use the same term, but in general we never hear it any more.

A good broad back is a fine thing, but broad backs and broad shoulders do not always go together. Some men have very long clavicles, and yet only have a narrow back. Still, the back is very easily built up, and as the back muscles become stronger they pull the shoulders back, making the bodily carriage more erect. One sure thing about the trapezius is that you cannot develop them fully without the aid of the latissimus dorsi muscles. I know you have been taught that shrugging the shoulders while holding a bar bell at arms' length across the thigh is a very good exercise. There is no doubt that it is, but you must always bear in mind that because this muscle has a threefold origin, it cannot be fully developed from one angle or by one exercise. We find that by bridging and shrugging, the trapezius is developed from two angles. The way this muscle works is in this fashion: The upper fibers elevate the shoulder girdle, and the lower fibers pulling on the base of the spine of the scapula depress the vertebral margin. These two movements result in a rotation of the shoulder blade. The main action is to draw the scapula backwards and upwards, like drawing the shoulders back, and raising the arms overhead. Now, this movement being understood, let us figure which exercise will give the best results. Shrugging the shoulders we will retain as one good exercise, but I am satisfied it does not fulfill all of our requirements. Still, pressing a bar bell overhead was always considered good. Well, I only rate it as being fair, but I do not lose track of the existence of this muscle being vitally important in raising objects overhead. At the same time, we all know that the back is stronger than the arms. Then our object should be to develop the back muscles by movements that will give them their fullest contraction. Pressing a bar bell off the chest to arms' length involves the operation of many muscles, but as the arms are naturally carried forward, the trapezius muscles are not fully contracted. Now if you place the bar-bell across the back of the neck, resting upon the shoulders, and by standing perfectly erect, begin to press the bar-bell to arms' length, you will find an altogether different action is brought upon the trapezius muscles. They will bulge more.

At one time bar-bell users trained considerably with dumb-bells, but at the present time dumb-bells and kettle-bells are seldom used. Perhaps you may not think so, but to press a pair of dumb-bells to arms' length overhead, is much more difficult than pressing a bar bell, and this is even so of the jerk. If you have any doubt about it, and you are able to jerk one hundred and fifty pounds overhead with both hands, just load up a pair of dumb-bells to seventy-five pounds each and try to jerk them. You will find it much harder. If, using a bar-bell, you are able to jerk two hundred pounds overhead, it is doubtful if you can jerk the same weight with dumb-bells. When you get up to heavy weights, from two hundred pounds up, you will find that kettle weights are even harder to handle than dumb-bells. One reason is, that one arm is weaker than the other, and the division of weight makes the weaker arm do its full share of the work without the aid of the stronger arm.

A good exercise practiced with kettle bells is pressing each one alternately from the shoulder to arms' length overhead, but a better one is practiced by standing erect with a dumb-bell in each hand, hanging by the side, with the feet together and body erect. With a pure arm movement, curl one dumb-bell to the shoulder, and press overhead. As you begin to lower this overhead dumbbell, curl the other and press it aloft. Keep on raising each one after the other from the side and going overhead, in a continuous movement. By this I mean, you must not stop at the shoulder, neither when going up or when coming down. A variation of this exercise can be done using both dumb-bells at once. Curl them to the shoulder and press them simultaneously. These full movements completely employ all the trapezius muscle in all its movements of full contraction. Also, the latissimus dorsi muscle is largely called into action. As these muscles grow they deepen the mass of muscle that forms on the back, but if you have a craving to broaden the shoulders you will be obliged to employ different methods. This increase must be supplied by the latissimus dorsi muscles. As I have stated in other chapters, these broad muscles are attached to the biceptial groove of the upper arm, and any movement that draws the arm forward, naturally involves these muscles. Therefore, it stands to reason that the greater the resistance that draws the arms forward the greater the contraction that will be required to pull the arm backward. If you pull a bar bell to the chest off the floor, you will feel a great spreading of the shoulders as the latissimus dorsi comes into play. I was always very particular about the way I performed this movement, as I realized the value of the exercise, but it does not take any close figuring to understand why these muscles, being so large, must be given a great deal of resistance. A twenty-five-pound bar bell or even a fifty-pound bar bell is too light for the average man. He is capable of handling more, and must if he wants the results. The general way to practice this exercise was with the feet apart, legs straight and the body bent over, not quite at right angles to the waist; but in my quest to secure the position that would give the latissimus dorsi their best workout, I found that by bending the knees a little I was able to handle more weight, and the action was brought more directly upon the right muscles. By the other method too much effort is thrown upon the small of the back, due to the fact that the body cannot be so correctly centralized as it is when the knees are bent a little. Still, you may say it is giving the latissimus dorsi muscles action in the lumbar region. I certainly agree, but muscular activity in that region is not going to broaden the shoulders. The main effect of the exercise is absorbed too low down. It is the pull given by the arms, and the effect it creates upon the latissimus dorsi muscles in its process of insertion on the humerus, that is going to do the thing for us. When I take up my position to commence this exercise, I always allow the bar bell to hang at arms' length. You know you can hold a weight at arms' length, and you can allow it to hang at arms' length. The difference is that by holding, the muscles are tensed, while in the hang no muscular tension is required. Just pick the bar bell off the floor, about an inch, and allow it to hang in the arms a few moments. You will feel a drag upon the shoulders which spreads them to their fullest extent, then slowly pull the bell towards the chest. See that the elbows are pointed outwards, so that they are on a level with the shoulders at the finish of the exercise. You will feel the value of the bent knees, as the leg muscles come into action to resist the pulling forward tendency of the back. More weight can be handled this way and a better balance secured with the effort borne at the right place. As the weight is lowered, I never allow it to touch the floor, but always clear by about an inch, relaxing the muscular contraction at the hang, so all the possible pull is brought upon the shoulders. You will find that where you make twelve repetitions in the ordinary movement, you will be lucky to make nine in this more effective way; but the results are a hundred per cent, better. Yet another mighty good back broadener is a variation of the last exercise. Instead of a bar bell use a pair of dumb-bells. Place them between the feet and pull them separately to the chest. Don't make the mistake of pulling them to the waist and think that that movement is correct, or just as good. It is a lazy way of practicing either of these two exercises.

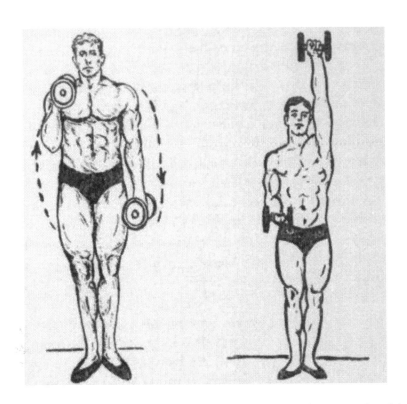

In the last named exercise I do not mean that you should pull one dumb-bell to the chest a number of times first. Let each hang in the hands at the same time, and alternately bring each one to the chest as many times as you feel comfortably able. Try it out with a pair of thirty-five-pound dumb-bells, and see that the elbow of each arm is always pointed well outwards so that all the possible spread is given to the shoulders.

I feel that we should consider the deltoids in this chapter, as they form part of the shoulder girdle and play an important part in shoulder construction, as well as enhancing the physical appearance. If you want to find out just how good your deltoids look, stand in front of the mirror in a relaxed pose. The chances are that the shoulders are going to have a slope that will be magnified by the lack of the fleshy mound which should appear at the extreme end of the collar-bone. To make sure that you are not being deceived, hold your arms out at full stretch, in a straight line with the shoulders, then clench the fists and bend the forearm on the upper arm. If these muscles are in a developed state, they will have a great fullness that will seem to have a cup shape. Undeveloped, they will be flat, and the biceps will have a bulkier appearance by contrast. The deltoid makes for the prominence of the shoulder, and derives its name from the fourth letter of the Greek alphabet, delta, because this muscle is shaped like the tri-angular formation of that letter. It has a threefold attachment on the shoulder blade, the collar-bone, and the humerus bone. Its operating duties are to lift the arm horizontally with the shoulder, sideways and in front. The fibers of this muscle are not as finely woven as those found in most other muscles. Its structure is really very coarse. The developing process of this muscle requires a little more careful consideration than any other muscle in the body, not because it is a weaker muscle, but because the methods of exercise include a certain leverage not found anywhere else, and the exerciser is apt to not consider this point when laying out his routine.

The muscular principles of leverage are just the same as the mechanical principles involved in raising a stone with a stick. If you have a long lever against a heavy object, you are going to move it easier, but if you change your point of leverage, taking only a short hold with the hands and allowing the heavy object to be at the long end of the stick, it is going to be a harder task to accomplish. That is just what the deltoids are up against. The kettle- weight, or any other object you are using, is at the farthest end of the leverage po.int, as against a shorter control, and that is why we cannot hold much weight at arms' length in a line with the shoulder. But, if you bend your arm at the elbow and allow the hand to come close up to the chest, you will be able to handle twice as much weight as at arms' length, because the leverage is shortened and the advantage is more with the deltoid. So, when you start to develop the deltoid muscle, do not allow your ambitions to run away with you and imagine that you can handle more weight than you are able. Start out easily.

Most of the exercises for the deltoids are best performed with kettle weights. The crucifix is probably the most popular exercise. The manner in which most exercise fans perform the crucifix is something like this. Taking a kettle bell in each hand, they curl them to the shoulders, and from this point they thrust the arms out horizontally with the shoulders, with the palms of the hands held up. It is not much of an exercise, and seldom registers any great degree of deltoid growth. The movement is too isolated. It causes the muscle to tense rather than give them a full contraction. As I have always remarked, if you want to get the most out of your muscles, you will have to give them full contraction, which means the same exercise must give them equally full extension. Therefore, the best movement is to commence with the hands hanging by the side, and without leaning backwards, raise the kettle bell until they are in a straight line with the shoulders, and then lower them. This exercise can be performed with variations, such as raising the arms from the side with the palms of the hands turned down, then with the palms turned up. In doing any of these movements try and shorten the length of leverage; when you raise the kettle bells with the palms turned up, bend the hand at the wrist towards the shoulder. With palms down, bend the hand at the wrist back on the forearm towards the shoulder. Perform the crucifix, or muscling out exercise, lowering the weights from above as well as raising from below. Also, lower them from above without a stop until the kettle bells hang at arms' length by the sides, then raise back to arms' length overhead, always keeping the arms straight. Raise the weights alternately as well as simultaneously, from the front as well as the sides, and your deltoids will quickly take on both shape and size that will add to the breadth of the shoulders. Muscling out was a great practice at one time, and I can well remember the time when this practice was very popular with laymen and professionals.

In the highlands of Scotland, throwing the shoulder stone was a great pastime, and it is one of the most ancient sports known to history. I have often visited the glen where a certain stone was kept for that purpose. This sport was often combined with muscling out, but this was much easier than holding out a ring weight. A stone weighing from forty pounds up is often large, although that depends a lot upon the composition of the stone, as some are much heavier than others. However, they generally looked for a flat stone, which rested as much on the forearm as the flat of the hand. The French used block weights considerably. I remember that most of their block weights are more oblong than those we use, and part of the block weight rested on the forearm, too. Our block weight is much like the English block weight, the only difference being that ours weigh fifty pounds and the English block weight is fifty-six pounds. Nearly every man I ever saw with a fine flat back, and broad shoulders, had a finely shaped pair of deltoids, and if you practice the exercises I have described in this chapter, you will quickly acquire the carriage of a grenadier, with the backbone of a real God-made man.

CHAPTER XV
SOME FASCINATING FACTS AND FIGURES

Figures to every man who is interested in the sport of weight lifting have the same fascinating interest that time has to the runner, height to the pole vaulter, and distance to the shot-putter and hammer thrower. A thrill is evidenced when an exceptionally good record is equaled or broken. Conquest is that for which everybody thirsts. The spectators applaud to see the athlete conquer. No matter how our customs change, the world remains the same in that one respect. We always have a passion to surpass. During the last few years the sport of weight lifting has been subject to a greater upheaval of surpassed marks than any other sport. It is not so long ago that this sport was looked upon as the special sport of just two or three countries. Now the whole world embraces it. Many experts in the sport has seen fit to say that certain marks could never be reached, certain records could never be equaled, and that the limit was almost reached on other lifts. Those prophecies have vanished like the records they embraced, with the possible exception of a few. The only reason that few stand is that the lifts on which the records are held are not used as frequently any more, in competition. Time was when the continental style of lifting was all the thing, whereby a weight or weights were taken to the shoulders in two or more movements, and then jerked or pushed overhead.

Personally, I was very sorry to see the two hands continental jerk pass away, for it robbed us of our most powerful men. I still feel that if the International Federation of Weight Lifters would accept five lifts for competition, and include the two hands continental, the results would be better all around. This would give the "continental" style lifter a chance, and the "clean" lifter would still have the balance of lifts in his favor, although the battle would be harder. I base my argument upon the knowledge that both layman and athlete are most interested in the largest poundage that one man can lift. For example, any of us would have a very hard job to convince another person that Rigoulot was as strong a man as Swoboda. The Frenchman is a clean lifter, pure and simple, with no inference ever made that he could lift as much, or more, in the continental style. It is doubtful if he can. His best lift is given as three hundred and seventy-six pounds in the two hands clean, with Swoboda lifting four hundred and twenty-two pounds in the two hands continental. I have been informed by quite a few European lifters who were personally acquainted with the Vienna butcher and his lifts, that he had jerked to arms' length from the shoulders the immense total of four hundred and thirty-eight pounds. He was helped with the weight to the shoulder, but they positively swear that, unaided, he jerked it, and held it aloft.

Most people would want to know how Rigoulot could be as strong,—or stronger, according to the style employed—than Swoboda. I know it would be a waste of time to argue. However, there is no comparison in their pressing ability. Swoboda has a record of three hundred and eleven pounds against Rigoulot's press of two hundred and twenty-three pounds. I feel quite sure that a back bend was used in the first place, although I cannot see such a huge man as Swoboda being capable of bending more than is allowed in the French style. The ruling on the French style has been changed somewhat. The judges agree it is not legal to bend in a press, but it is permissible to bend back as far as the lifter desires, prior to the press. This may sound a little complicated, but what they mean is that the lifter can bend back when the weight is at the shoulder, but the body is not allowed to bend while the lift is in progress. Rigoulot made that poundage of two hundred and twenty-three pounds in his match with Cadine, the latter only making one hundred and ninety-eight pounds. I should also say that the clean lift by Rigoulot is not official; his official lift is three hundred and sixty-four pounds. Just the same, Swoboda's four hundred and thirty-eight pounds jerk is unofficial, but we all know that lifters can acquire excellent form while training which has enabled them to totally eclipse many of their best public performances. Nevertheless, the marks that have been set in training are just as honest as when performed in competition. Therefore, it is my intention to give you all the facts and figures that I know of, whether they were done in training or in competition, just as long as they are honest. This being perfectly understood, I will continue with my comparisons. The next great two-handed lifter was the other wonderful Vienna lifter, Josef Steinbach. He stood five feet nine and a half inches and scaled about two hundred and forty-seven pounds. From the shoulder he jerked three hundred and eighty and a quarter pounds twice to arms' length, and in one jerk he did three hundred and ninety pounds, which puts him close to Swoboda. Yet, I am pretty sure that Herman Gorner could do as well, if not better. This South African German has taken to the shoulders in two movements a four hundred and forty and a half-pound bar bell without any aid, a feat which exceeds Swoboda's. However, he did not jerk it aloft. But, stop and figure what he might be capable of in a two hands continental jerk, when I tell you that he has jerked overhead from behind the neck three hundred and ninety-seven pounds in living weight. Officially, he is only a half pound behind Rigoulot's official record performance, with three hundred and sixty-three and a half pounds, but as we see, he is capable of eclipsing them all, as proven by his jerk from behind the neck. Then we have Alzin of France, who cleans over three hundred and sixty pounds, and is considered even greater in the continental style, which no doubt he is, because of his great weight. Cadine goes over three hundred and fifty pounds, and Saxon without any effort did a two hands clean in New York of three hundred and fifty-eight pounds. Henry Steinborn has cleaned and jerked on several occasions three hundred and fifty pounds. I saw him jerk the three hundred and fifty pounds three times in succession at Professor Attila's gymnasium. On another occasion, at Siegmund Klein s gymnasium, I saw him jerk three hundred and seventy pounds. Karl Moerke cleans over three hundred and fifty-three pounds. And in the continental style I have his picture snapped as he jerked aloft three hundred and seventy-five pounds. Wilhelm Tureck, another Austrian, who won the world's title in 1898, raised three hundred and fifty-five pounds. While no record mentioned whether this was a clean lift or not, yet I am inclined to believe it was not, as they never "cleaned" in those days. All this goes to show that our present day crop of strength athletes can compare very favorably with the great heroes of the past, especially if you consider body weight in the comparison. Cadine weighs less than two hundred pounds, at a height of five feet six inches. Rigoulot makes two hundred and sixteen pounds and stands five feet seven and a half inches. Steinborn makes two hundred pounds, while Moerke weighs about two hundred and twenty pounds and stands only five feet two inches, with Gorner the heaviest, weighing two hundred and forty-five pounds. He is also the tallest, being over six feet tall. All the older men, like Cyr, Barre, and Swoboda, went three hundred pounds and over, with Steinbach and Tureck about two hundred and fifty pounds. Andreas Maier, the German, was the lightest of the big men of twenty years ago, and incidentally one of the best. He stood five feet seven inches and weighed one hundred and ninety-six pounds, but he had a continental jerk record of three hundred and sixty-two pounds and in the clean style he made the first German record that he set at three hundred and eleven pounds. So far, we find that the heaviest weight gotten overhead in the two hands jerk goes to Swoboda and Gorner. Now there is another two- handed lift, known as the two hands anyhow, in which a man can employ any method at all in order to stand erect, while the weights are held overhead in both hands. Arthur Saxon, who was so mighty in the bent press, raised the total combined weight of four hundred and forty-eight pounds. From various quarters I have heard this lift scouted, simply because Saxon employed the bent press. That is both foolish and unfair, but just to see how good this Teuton was we will cut out that lift, where the bent press was employed, so we can satisfy all concerned and prove the great strength of Arthur Saxon. Three hundred and eleven pounds in the two hands clean was nothing to him; more than a dozen times when he had jerked it overhead, he gave his onlookers a little idea of how contemptuously he held that poundage by tossing the weight into one hand, and throwing it back to the other. At such a time he was seen to throw the weight into one hand, and then lean over and pick a one hundred and twelve-pound kettle weight off the floor with the other hand, and press aloft, making a total poundage of four hundred and twenty-three pounds. This, you must understand, was impromptu lifting, just for exhibition purposes. Later he did four hundred and forty- eight pounds officially. In comparison with this, we find Herman Gorner, a man who never makes a bent press, raising the enormous weight of four hundred and forty and three-quarter pounds. Personally, I think that Gorner is the most powerful man of all times. On a set of ten lifts I believe he would have beaten any of the giants of the past when they were at their best, as safely as he will any of the present luminaries. It is a well known fact that he is the only athlete who over a period of fifteen years could be relied upon to do over three hundred and thirty pounds in a two hands clean without warming up.

Unlike most "clean" lifters, Gorner is a fine press lifter, although it seems none of them can come near to the great Steinbach on such lifts. In November of 1907, in Vienna, he is credited with performing a two hands push of three hundred and eighty-six and seven-eighths pounds. Two years previously he had pressed a bar bell of two hundred and eighty-five pounds, while standing with the heels together, and in a continental press he claims three hundred and thirty-five pounds. But the king of all, in the two hands military press, is Karl Witzelsberger, another Austrian, of two hundred and thirty-eight pounds, who is given credit for three hundred pounds. Then there is his two hands jerk of three hundred and seventy-eight pounds to be considered, which goes to show that like Steinbach, Gorner, Alzin and Rigoulot, he is a versatile lifter. In other words, he combines all- round ability; speed with power. With dumb-bells he was a fine lifter, and along with Steinbach he seems to stand among the foremost. Dumb- bell lifting is a real test of strength. The divided poundage develops an awkwardness that takes real manpower to overcome. Witzelsberger came only five pounds behind Steinbach's record of three hundred and thirty-five pounds in the two dumb-bells jerk. I have invariably found that a good press lifter is a good dumb-bell lifter, and vice versa. At the present time dumb-bell lifting is not practiced much outside of Canada, where Giroux reigns supreme in these lifts, and has successfully lifted two hundred and seventy- eight pounds in what was termed a two dumb-bells jerk. It looked more like a press to me. An interesting truth is that Giroux just heaves his upper body at the weight in all his jerk lifts, and finishes them all by pressing the weight out with his arms. Hector DeCarrie was great at jerking dumb- bells, but pride of place at the present time goes to Gorner, who has done three hundred and thirty and a half pounds, which makes him a close contender for Steinbach's record. Cyr and Barre were in the three hundred-pound class when it came to tossing around dumb-bells, and they were also great press men. It is a pity we have no record of what Sergi Moor, the Russian lifter, could do with dumb-bells. He only weighed one hundred and ninety pounds, but they gave him credit for a two handed bar bell push of three hundred and nineteen and a half pounds. He must have been a freak to be able to push such an enormous poundage to arms' length at so light a bodyweight, I never heard what he could do in any other lift. Arthur Saxon has a record of two hundred and sixty-nine pounds in a Military Press, but I am inclined to believe Gorner is going to beat it. The Military Press of two hundred and forty-two and a half pounds was made a long while ago by Herman, and just recently I received a photo showing Gorner making an impromptu push with two hundred and sixty pounds, at that he was fully dressed except for his coat, as he stood ankle deep in loose sand. Of course, there is a lot of difference in a push and a military press, but believe me, any man who can stand up to a strange, solid type bar bell with dumbbells tied on to it to make up the weight, and even keep his collar on, can military press the same weight. Why! he had no trouble making a press of two hundred and seventy-three and a half pounds, which goes to show how he is improving. He is one lifter who has kept abreast of the times. When the weight lifting federation decided that for the future only clean lifts would govern the sport of lifting weights, he was fully capable to comply with the change, whereas men like Swoboda were not, due to their extreme bulk. It seems peculiar that a man will allow himself to fall into a groove in lifting. I find that some of them figure like this, "Well, I've done that style of lifting all my life, and I'm not good at the other styles, so what is the use of me bothering anymore." It is just like trying to persuade some hundred-yard men to try two hundred and twenty yards. They think the change is too much. That is foolish. One time I was watching Giroux lift and I noticed how high he pulled the weights in that he pressed, so I said to him, "Listen Arthur, see how high you can pull that weight without finishing with a press." He commenced with two hundred and thirty pounds and found it a little difficult, then as he got better accustomed to what he was supposed to do, he finally snatched two hundred and fifty -six pounds. He did not make those fast dips as an aid, that we find practiced by the energetic skillful lifter, for two reasons. In the first place, he is very heavy, and secondly, he is a phlegmatic type of athlete. What he lacked in dynamic energy as displayed by men like Rigoulot, Cadine, and Stein- born, he made up by a greater power that can apply itself forcibly in a longer physical resistance against gravitation. Now if he can do it, so can the others. However, it is no use complaining because they did not adjust themselves, for it takes all kinds of people to make a world.

The British lifters have always followed the "clean" lifts, but they have never produced any remarkable big men in that style. Therefore, I do not believe it was any influence of theirs that swung the sport of weight lifting. It might have been the desire to see the joint record held by Cyr and Barre of three hundred and forty-seven pounds, effaced from the record sheets. They certainly had a great deal of respect for Cyr. However, it could have been one of many other reasons, but I give credit to Louis Vasseur, the famous French veteran, for creating the first interest in fast lifting. This wonderful lifter just dazzled the Parisians with his vital strength. His first great achievement was his two arm snatch of two hundred and forty-nine pounds performed at the low bodyweight of one hundred and eighty-nine pounds. He followed this with a brilliant one hand snatch of two hundred and nine and a half pounds, which remained a world's record for many years. Tromp Van Diggelen, a man who has been one of the great pillars of this sport, and incidentally the man who produced Max

Sick and Herman Gorner, told me that he had seen Vasseur snatch two hundred and twenty- two pounds, which is corroborated by others who have witnessed the same feat. Then commenced the interest in clean jerks, snatches and swings, which gradually grew in popularity until they monopolized the whole field. We find the older veteran, Pierre Bonnes, forging ahead in the two hands snatch with two hundred and fifty-four pounds, and young Maurice De Riaz, the Swiss athlete, when not much more than a middleweight, snatching with two hands two hundred and nine and a half pounds. His brother, Emile, came along in the professional ranks and made a left hand snatch record of one hundred ninety-two and a half pounds. He also made the first left hand swing record with the same poundage of one hundred ninety- two and a half pounds. Then Jean François Le Breton equaled Arthur Saxon's right hand swing with two hundred pounds, which was followed by Heinrich Rondi with a one hand snatch of two hundred and four pounds. This same young man began to make things interesting by showing that he could do other things as well as snatch. Just to prove it, he made a two hands push with two hundred and eighty-six and a half pounds, and jerked three hundred and thirty and a half pounds. A new type of athlete came forward along with the "clean" method of lifting. Instead of the human colossus, there appeared men with size and form'. Men with godlike proportions, and muscles that spread their separations over the entire physique, like the giant roots of a fig tree. They combined the three physical graces, shape, size and strength. They crashed into the limelight to breathe a new inspiration. It looked to me as though it was a trick of fate that had taken these children from their Titian cradle, to disprove the old prejudices and fallacies, that only men of bulk with cart-horse proportions and density could lift weights. The clean cut Henry Steinborn was one of them. At one event he crashed the two hands clean and jerk record of the ponderous Cyr and Barre into the past by lifting three hundred and fifty-three pounds, and beat the official right hand snatch of Vasseur with a lift of two hundred and fifteen pounds, to be followed by a record in training that beat Louis Vasseur's unofficial two hundred and twenty-two pound snatch record, with two hundred and thirty pounds. Then the battle began, first Cadine, then Rigoulot, then Strassburger, all racing for the laurels of victory. The laurels were finally hung on the neck of Rigoulot, only to be snatched away by the powerful Gorner on the total of ten lifts. Already, Alzin of Marseilles has badly beaten the totals of Cadine and Rigoulot, and he is crowding Gorner hard, so where it will all end I do not know. A long while ago, Alfred Alzin made a two hands snatch with two hundred and fifty-six and a half pounds, and a two hands continental jerk with three hundred and seventy-nine pounds. On the dead lift, with either one or two hands, Gorner has them all so badly swamped that no matter how they try, they cannot score over him. Not long ago, Paris was stirred by the fact that Cadine had succeeded in lifting the huge, thick handled bar bell that once belonged to Louis Uni (Apollon). Up to that time it had defied the efforts of all the best strength athletes of every nation. The total poundage was given out as about six hundred pounds. Just before that, Cadine made a new record of five hundred and eighty-nine pounds, which scrapped Leon Verhaert's five hundred and fifty-seven pound record of years' standing.

Later, at the Halterophile Club in Paris, he raised with two hands six hundred and twenty-pounds. This was claimed as a world's record, but Giroux in Philadelphia about the same time, raised in fine style six hundred and fifty pounds. Then, like a bolt from the blue, came Gorner's smashing two hands dead lift record of seven hundred ninety three and three quarter pounds. In the meantime, Cadine had set up a new one hand record with about four hundred and nineteen pounds, and a little less than four hundred pounds with the left hand. The left hand record was beaten by the Boston veteran middleweight, John Y. Smith, who raised in great style four hundred pounds, and was just a little unfortunate in not beating the Frenchman's right hand record by six pounds. Despite his fifty-nine years of age, he raised four hundred and ten pounds. By this time we had become accustomed to the South African's great two hand dead lift, when into my office comes another bomb shell certifying that Gorner had made a new one hand dead lift record of seven hundred and twenty- seven and a quarter pounds. The lift is verified officially. Well, it made me smile, simply because this powerful Boer is only proving my prophesies of the lifts that I stated would be accomplished before many years had gone by. I do not become surprised at anything else I hear that this South African member of the A. C. W. L. A. performs. When I received the report of his miraculous right hand swing of two hundred and twenty and a half pounds, and his left hand swing of two hundred and three and three quarter pounds, I simply paid my tribute to this mighty son of Vulcan. His wonderful snatch of two hundred and seventy-five and a half pounds was passed by Rigoulot with a terrific lift of two hundred and seventy-seven pounds.

About the same time at the Club Athletique des Boulets in Paris, the same young Poilu beat the dumb-bell snatch record of Maurice DeRiaz, which stood at two hundred and two pounds by adding four more pounds to the total. With a dumb-bell it is a most marvelous performance. Still, it surprises me a little how low some of them remain on the press, although Rigoulot is improving fast. None of them can equal most of the American and Canadian lifters. Giroux does two hundred and fifty-six pounds in the European style, and in the strict military style, Steinborn does two hundred and thirty pounds, and Moerke two hundred and forty-two pounds, while recently I succeeded with two hundred and forty-five pounds. Of course, Gorner is top dog in this lift as previously stated, and I feel sure our present day strength athletes will some day surpass the records of the former athletes, as completely on this lift as any other, with the possible exception of the lift by Steinbach. Socrates Temeli, of Roumania, made a bar bell press of two hundred and eighty- six and three quarter pounds, and he has a Continental jerk record of three hundred seventy and a half pounds. However, it must not be forgotten that the press and push lifters, performed by our present time lifters, were all taken in clean to the shoulders in one movement. Making this comparison, I am afraid many of the old timers' records have already fallen. I know that I can press far more than I can clean. Then there is Joe Nordquest, who is handicapped by the loss of one leg, but he has pressed two hundred and fifty-six pounds. On all round lifting the modern lifter is far ahead.

The one hand clean and jerk was another sticker for the old time lifters, who did not seem to be able to go far with it. We find the pioneer of energetic lifts, Louis Vasseur, setting up the first right hand clean with two hundred and thirty pounds, and great little Maurice DeRiaz, swinging into line with two hundred twenty-three and three quarter pounds, officially. Later, he performed in the presence of many notable athletes a one hand clean of two hundred and forty-five pounds. George Hackenschmidt did two hundred thirty-one pounds, when only a boy, and G. Lassartesse did two hundred and twenty-five pounds. So far, H. Gaessler, of Germany, seems to have it on them all in this lift, as he is given credit for two hundred fifty-one pounds, right hand, and two hundred twenty and a half pounds, left. Given competition, Gorner would wreck all these one hand clean and jerk records. He has taken to the shoulder with two hands a bar bell of two hundred sixty- four and a half pounds, and from there, he jerked the weight to arms' length with the right arm only. I was told that Arthur Saxon had performed around two hundred and sixty pounds in a one hand clean and jerk, which is not to be doubted. The one hand military press that was set up by Arthur Saxon at one hundred twenty-six pounds has been always considered to be the greatest genuine military press ever made. I have not lost sight of the wonderful mark set up by Karl Witzelsberger of one hundred sixty-two pounds, nor the one hundred fifty-eight pound press by Barre, and LaVallee with his one hundred sixty-five pound record, but it is generally conceded that these athletes bent slightly, even though the legs were kept locked. Of course, they did not bend far, but two inches in this lift means a lot, as you all know. It is sufficient to relieve the pressure at the most difficult part of the lift, anyhow, Jean François Le Breton succeeded with one hundred twenty-four pounds in the perfect style, as we understand it, and I have seen Giroux do one hundred thirty-eight pounds French style. In the real military style, I could always win from him. Quite contrary to the general belief, a man who has trained himself to bend slightly in this one lift, finds it very difficult not to do so; while a man who has accustomed himself to the rigid style can perform either way. Josef Hofbeck, the one hundred and fifty-four pound Austrian crack, has a record of one hundred twenty-three and a half pounds in the European style. It is impossible to believe that anything else but a slight bend was employed, for no one would believe that a one hundred and fifty-four pound man could surpass a man like Gorner, who makes a perfect one hand military of one hundred and twenty-one pounds. When I was much lighter than I am now, I found no difficulty in military pressing with one hand, French style, one hundred and thirty-six pounds, at the same time I held the record in strict military style with one hundred and ten pounds in my class. At the time I surpassed Arthur Saxon's record, performing one hundred twenty-seven and a half pounds, I could easily press one hundred and fifty pounds French style. It was the fact that I was so good on a one hand military press that made me so good on a one hand Continental press, in which lift I had done two hundred as a middleweight, a feat that stopped most of the heavyweights. Yet, there is a lot in how a man takes to a lift. We all pick on certain ones, and it is generally on those we do our best. The same thing happens with a football team, one man plays better in one part of the field than he does in another. Many people have often said to me that a certain lifter should be better at other lifts than he was, as compared with some of his best lifts. Quite often I have found the answer that the lifter did not like those certain lifts. Although I worked up fairly high on the bent press, yet I cared for that lift the least of any. Mention of the bent press will bring to your mind the thought that here is one lift I have overlooked. Such is not the case. I have only treated with the recognized standard lifts as used by all countries in competition. With the exception of Britain, the lift is never used in competition. Canada has the finest bent press men, at the present, but the lift is not included among the ten French Canadian Weight Lifting Federation Lifts. For many years weight lifters in America were measured more by their bent press ability than anything else. With the inception of the American Continental Weight Lifting Association we have gotten away from it, and although at the present time there is a thousand strength athletes following the sport of weight lifting, to everyone that lifted weights ten years ago, there were considerably more bent press men then, than now. This does not mean that I am prejudiced against the bent press. I think it is a very useful lift, but if we have to meet lifters of other countries on their sets of lifts, which are controlled by the International Federation of Weight Lifting, we would be foolish to concentrate on lifts that have no competitive value. On the other hand, we have developed a great number of lifts, in fact, more than the British, but this is more to keep a tabulation upon the many feats of strength of which an athlete is capable. They all go to help make a lifter more efficient, although the majority of them I look upon as exercises more than competitive lifts. However, we never include them in competition. The American strength lifter has developed an entirely different method of training and lifting than that of any other country. It is entirely our own, and the proof of its value is testified to by the marked strides we have made in the last two or three years. Our progress has been more rapid than that of any other nation. A few years ago, we were considered positive failures, but today the American strength athlete has wrested many of the world's records from the best Europeans on the standard lifts. This goes for professionals as well as amateurs. Within the ranks of the American Continental Weight Lifter's Association, a team could be formed fit to meet a team from any other country. We have everything from snatch lifters to finger lifters, two handed lifters to back lifters, and all top notchers.

Speaking of back lifters reminds me of the great back lift by Louis Cyr, which stood at three thousand six hundred and fifty-three pounds, but it is not so well known that his great partner, Horace Barre, made a back lift of three thousand eight hundred and ninety pounds, and it is less known that LaVallee actually lifted four thousand pounds. Although I always believe that Warren Lincoln Travis would lift the coveted poundage of two tons if he was extended in competition. Certainly he has come closer to it than any other man. French Canada once could boast of a great woman back lifter, Madame Cloutier, and in a match with Flossie La Blanche she made a back lift of twenty-five hundred pounds. Yet our interest will always be centered around the bar bell and dumb-bell lifters, and some day we are going to see Alzin, Gorner and Rigoulot brought together, then the records will fly.

The future is full of promise, because the present time weight lifter possesses a greater abundance of speed and energy coupled to his strength. He tackles his proposition with all the conserved power of a machine gun. That is why we see men weighing one hundred pounds lighter than Louis Cyr, lifting a greater poundage than the great Louis ever did in his palmiest days in the two hands clean and jerk.

CHAPTER XVI
How to Develop Superb Hips and Thighs

If I were to be asked, which are the muscles to which muscle builders pay the least attention, I would say the muscles of the legs. For every one physical culturist that I see with a pair of well built legs, I see fifty without them. It is also a fact, that the majority of people I meet who possess good legs were aided by nature in the first place. Naturally, development was not very hard for them to acquire. Honestly, I admire a man who has earned his leg development. I know just what he has gone through. The knowledge that the average exercise fan has at his command for promoting the growth of these various muscles is very meager, which means that he has had to go through a lot of tortuous work in order to succeed, as well as call upon all the reserves of his will power.

It is very common to see a splendid upper body development spoiled by a pair of spindly legs, and the trouble is, that the average exercise fan does not wake up until he is made to feel very conscious of the fact.

You will always hear the same old worn out alibi when you ask them why they did not spend an equal amount of time upon developing their legs:—"I do exercise them, but they just won't grow." Well, let us agree on the point that they all do a certain amount of training according to their knowledge, and let us see just about how much they are likely to do. Ninety percent are limited by just practicing the squat, or deep knee bend. Another five percent add the exercise, which is a variation of the Kennedy Lift. In this movement the position is taken astride a bar bell and the bar is grasped with one hand in front of the body and the other hand behind. Standing erect, only a slight bend of the knees is made a number of times. The remaining five percent have either developed some exercise movements of their own, or have received some expert coaching. It is among this last quota that you will find the few who have actually earned their leg muscles. Consequently, we find the majority of body culturists using only two exercises at the most. Compare these two with the number of movements employed for arm development. There is no comparison at all. If as much time was spent on proportioning the legs as is spent upon the biceps, we would certainly see better legs. It is actually the craze for big biceps and chest muscles that absorbs most of a student's exercise period, which has brought about the spindly leg condition.

It is my intention to devote this article entirely to the thighs, which will compel the including of the hips by reason of their co-operative existence. To a certain extent the calf muscles are brought into action by these same movements, but not enough to guarantee any amount of muscular growth.

The mere suggestion of an exercise without an explanation, is like putting a ship to sea without a rudder. It sails, but gets nowhere, and to name the muscles is not sufficient. We have to go much deeper. We have to find out just why that muscle is there; how it operates; or whether it operates best alone, or in conjunction with another muscle. Then we have something on which to work. This knowledge enables us to find out the best means of control in order to make muscles more subject to growth. Boiled down, we become acquainted with the cause, effect, and determination of the muscles and their growth.

Commencing with the front part of the thigh, which is properly known as the anterior aspect, we find that the Quadriceps Femoris is the chief muscle, and covers the major frontal portion. As the first part of the name implies, this muscle is fourfold. The name is significant of another fact, which testifies that these muscles work in one group.

Of course, many muscles work in groups, but nature adapted these particular four for actual co-ordination. They are capable of greater resistance because of their fourfold nature. Consequently, any exercise that involves the Quadriceps as a group, can safely be of a vigorous nature.

The Quadriceps have generally been explained as the triceps of the thighs. Not in the sense that this group is threefold, as the word triceps implies, but to illustrate the fact that the Quadriceps operates like the triceps of the arm. That is, it helps to straighten the leg. Yet, if you examine the anatomical construction of the front of the thigh, you will almost be led to believe that the Quadriceps is composed of three muscles. However, it is not, because the Rectus Femoris has a double tendinous origin. The word Rectus, explains to you that the muscle operates in erection, or straightening.

In fact, the Rectus Femoris is a very interesting twin muscle. It is a flexor of the hip joint. Therefore, any exercise that involves these twin muscles must necessarily employ the hip muscles. Under physical movement, the straight head acts when the movement begins, and the reflected head is tightened when the thigh becomes bent.

The parts of the Quadriceps extensor are supplied by separate branches of the Femoral nerve, which is the reason why the thigh muscles can operate in terrific movements of propulsion, where great nervous energy is required, such as speed racing and lifting heavy weights overhead quickly.

The Externus Vastus muscle, the one on the extreme outside of the thigh, is always the most noticeable on an athlete. It is the hump of muscle so easily discernible, about one-third of the distance up the thigh, which arcs outwards in one sweeping curve to the hip. Just tense your thigh by locking the knee tightly backwards, and you will see how it shapes itself. But this muscle is not entirely surfacial as the outward contour makes it appear. If you raise the leg to right angles with the body, you will notice a little hump of muscle about two inches long lying along the outside, at the extreme end of the thigh nearest the hip. This muscle is attached by a very long tendon that runs down the side of the thigh to the knee. It is under this muscle that the Externus Vastus finally loses itself. Raise your leg again and you will learn something more. Aside from the appearance of the little hump of muscle, you will notice that the Externus Vastus becomes so vigorously tensed that you can see it taper to its tendon.

Now let us get back to exercise. The squat or deep knee bend, whichever you want to call it, is generally practiced balanced upon the toes with the heels close together. I once read a statement that of the Quadriceps group, this exercise developed the Internus Vastus the most. But I disagree, and I will tell you why. I have noticed that this particular muscle is lacking in development with most of the indoor exercise fans. Even the majority of weight lifters do not show the pronounced development we would expect. It is the Rectus Femoris and the Externus Vastus that are the most prominent. But if you practice the deep knee bend with the feet flat on the floor pointed forwards, you will soon find that this bunch of muscle just above the knee cap, on the inside of the thigh, will grow rapidly, for this reason. With the heels together and the bodyweight balanced upon the ball of the feet, you cannot make as deep a squat, which is necessary to bring this muscle vigorously into action. It is always noticeable that strong men who finish their feats with a deep knee bend, have well formed Internus Vastus muscles. The Germans call it the Shenkel muscle, which means "a muscle of the shank." That is why I prefer a flat foot squat, because it brings the entire group of Quadriceps muscles into play at once, and does away with the necessity of a number of exercises that are not required. This again proves the fact that when you find the right exercise, where a natural group of muscles co-ordinate so powerfully, as in this case, you can secure better results.

However, we have more muscles to consider. For one, the little hump on the top outside of the thigh.

In most cases, the Externus Vastus start off with a sweeping arc, but instead of completing the curve, it becomes a straight line. Why? Well now, did you not learn something when you raised your leg to right angles with the body? Remember how this little muscle tensed, and you felt such a powerful contraction of the entire Externus Vastus? Perhaps you also noticed how insignificant the little mound of tissue was. Proof you have not exercised the muscle to promote any growth, but if you do, you will create an appearance when the thigh is tensed that will form a beautiful curve from where the Externus Vastus commences all the way up to the groin. This muscle is always highly developed in football kickers, because its action has a lot to do with raising the leg forward.

Just hitch your toes in the handle of a light kettle bell and raise the leg forward to right angles with the body. Keep the leg perfectly straight and don't lean backwards too far or bend the other knee too deeply. You will probably find it necessary to place one hand lightly on the back of a chair in order to control your balance. This is a fine developer.

Now we come to the last important muscle on the face of the thigh. The one that gives the thigh that fullness so pleasing to the sight. It is a long strip of muscle that is attached at the extreme height of the thigh on the outside, and crosses the top of the entire thigh to become fastened on the inside of the shin bone just below the knee. We call it the Sartorious, which means "The tailor's muscle." The Germans call it the "cutting" muscle. Both express the meaning adequately. The German version implies that is cuts across the others, but I like our interpretation best, as it seems to contain more. The abductor tendencies of this muscle is not as great as the Femoris, despite its great length. The Tailor's muscle is mostly employed in rotating the leg from side to side. Another of its great functioning qualities is the direct effect it has of supporting the Quadriceps muscle. I believe that from its capacity to act in this direction, it acquired its peculiar name. Anything special a tailor would do on his work, would naturally be as a better aid or support, or to give better service. His object would be to bind the material better. The Sartorious acts the same way. Something like a strap around a barrel, it straps around the Quadriceps muscles and holds them more powerfully together under vigorous movement. Stick your foot into the handle of the light kettle bell and again raise the foot to right angles. From this position move the leg from side to side as much as possible, but be sure to keep it straight.

I hope you have all this clearly fixed in your mind, and that my explanations have enlightened you a little more on these muscles. Of course, the muscles I have named do not constitute the whole mass of tissue on the front of the leg. There are others that lie beneath, but their action is guided entirely by the surfacial muscles we have just studied.

We have the muscles on the back of the thigh to consider. Because the muscle builder cannot see them without the aid of a mirror is the main reason why they are so badly neglected. Just stand in profile in front of the mirror, and you will surprise yourself. From the back of the knee up to the buttock muscle, there is apt to be a straight line where a fullness should exist. Remember, your thigh is not developed unless it can stand criticism from every angle. Coming back to the point, I will explain that the muscles on the back of the thighs are called the biceps because of their double origin. They contract and control the body as the knees become bent. No doubt the thought has come to your mind, if this is the case, why are they not as well developed as the muscles on the front of your thigh from practicing the squat. I used to wonder why their appearance was not improved more than it is from the various deep knee bending exercises, but by careful observation of pupils in practice, I found the reason. The average exercise fan makes the squat far too quickly to really employ the biceps to any extent. The real exertion lies in coming to the erect position, and this exertion is entirely taken care of by the Quadriceps muscles.

A very peculiar but interesting feature about the muscles of the front of the thigh and the back of the thigh is their relative pole of balance.

Strange as it may seem, I have never seen it explained, yet I have seen lots of field and weight lifting coaches scratch their head in consternation. To their mind the athlete had all the science down pat, and for the world they could see no reason for his lack of improvement. In shot- putting, throwing the hammer and lifting weights, the athlete appeared to secure enough crouch or dip. But, there was the trouble, they got too much crouch or dip. I have met a few coaches who recognized the fact, but could not explain the cause, which bolsters my argument that you must know why you do a thing.

When I see an athlete make too deep a knee bend in lifting a weight overhead or in shot-putting and broad and high jumping, I immediately, mentally register a failure. The cause is that he has traveled past the pole of balance. Strange as it may seem, to secure the best effect, only a light dip is required of two or three inches; if the athlete travels further the biceps secure the balance of power. The snap is taken out of the movement. If anything, the balance should be with the Quadriceps.

The concentrated effort from the waist up registers a great downward pressure before the up-heave is made, and where any amount of weight is employed the downward pressure is always greater. Of course, the better developed the thigh biceps, the better is this condition overcome.

I found that lying upon a table with a kettle bell hitched on each foot, and then curling the heels to the buttock, was an ideal exercise for these muscles. Some allow a person to sit on the soles of the feet and curl their bodyweight, but a person is not always handy, as are kettle bells.

This exercise has a fine effect on the calf and buttocks also. You will find, lying on the back with a weight balanced on the feet and pressed to straight legs, is also very good.

Of course there are many other exercises that have a good influence upon the thighs, but as the major part of body culturists practice within the confines of their room these other movements are out of the question. But, if you can get out where your opportunities are not so restricted, you would naturally find improvement more rapid.

The benefits of thigh exercise do not begin and finish with the increased proportions and bettered appearance. You will find that in nearly all thigh movements the buttock muscles are equally involved, and as the thighs
improve the buttocks become firmer and will take on a fullness that will magnify the contours of the thighs. In fact, there will be a considerable change in the hips, groin, lower back and abdomen that is well worth working for.

However, I will not go so far as to say the chest and upper back will be benefited in proportion. I don't believe it. In theory it may sound all right, but anatomically it can't be done.

A person with wide hips will develop the largest legs, as he has the natural construction. That is, he has more space to build upon and generally is possessed of greater concentrated energy. The small of his back is wider and the rope muscles on his back appear like huge twisting columns. The pit of his body is larger and this gives a greater space for the entire torso. Such men always have powerful vital organs.

The part of the spine that embraces the region of the hips is known as the sacrum. Its translation signifies that it forms a sacred area, which we know it does. All our procreative powers are contained in this region, which makes it the reception of our virile forces. The ancient sages of biblical days when referring to famous men of their time would explain their qualities as being due to the fact that they "sprung from the loins" of so and so. Their term was more correct than our present day assertion that so and so is a real "chip of the old block."

The floor of the pelvis is a natural foundation for the base of the spine and considerable support is given to the fixed spines of the sacrum region by the depth and breadth of the hip bones. If a man has wide hips he is bound to have good legs, and, as I have inferred, any exercise that operates the thigh muscles brings into action the powerful buttock muscles. Have you noticed when you went to push against an object how these big muscles tightened up? The same thing happens if you resist somebody who seeks to push you away. These muscles contract very vigorously when a person bends backwards, as he pushes some object overhead. An exercise fan feels the resistance in all two-arm push and press exercises. I remember when I was making records in these lifts how many of my friends would remark that it was my great arm and back strength that enabled me to do so well. They were surprised when I explained to them that the whole secret of that lift was in the support I received from the buttock muscles. They were my support, and I could feel the bolstering effect upon the small of the back. Their tension helped to keep the knees locked, which is extremely important, for as the battle is fought to pass the sticking point in raising the weight aloft, the pressure upon the legs is greatest, and the least relaxation of tension at the knees will spoil the lift. As I referred in a previous chapter that years ago a favorite supporting feat of professional performers was to do what was termed a hip support. How they had a belt that fit loosely over the hips with a hook and chain attachment that passed through the platform on which they stood, to be fastened onto the supports of a platform underneath. On the platform were horses or a number of people. The lower platform was lowered (not always lifted) until the whole platform with the people on it would be suspended, supported by the strong man's hips. To make the feat more impressive, the lifter would press overhead a bar bell, or else hold kettle weights out at arms' length level with the shoulders in a crucifix. Then by a mouthpiece he would sustain the weight of some other heavy object. This feat is not nearly as hard as it looks, although it certainly requires strength: The main thing is to keep the knees locked against the great downward pressure. So you see, it is a great asset to have good hips from a physical standpoint as well as on account of the organic strength they control.

I often feel that the more we know about these facts the richer we become. We are taught to realize more than ever the efficacy of exercise. Observation and analysis teach us many interesting things.

My life has been spent among athletes of every form and no one has had any better opportunity of noting the effects of exercise and sport than I have had. Shot-putters, hammer throwers and sprint racers have the finest legs among field athletes. But I have noticed that it is only since the crouch start has been practiced among sprint racers that they have acquired an all-round thigh development. The old-time standing-up start never seemed to have much effect upon the Internus Vastus. Jumpers generally have good thighs, but none of these field athletes show the development in their upper body that some imagine. Shot-putters and hammer throwers naturally have the more powerful physique. Yet, they all fall short of the muscle builder. The latter studies his physique more thoroughly and seeks to perfect his proportions as well as to increase them. The sportsman runs, jumps or throws the hammer just for the love of the sport, and mostly train to master the science of his particular sport. As a rule, he is not interested in development, which is all wrong. I have increased the ability of many field athletes from constructional exercise. A body culturist is the best all-round athlete because he perfects his whole body. He is interested in harmonious development, which after all, is the only thing that counts.

The biggest fault I have against the home exercise fan is that he will fall into such unpardonable hit-and-miss habits. Just consider the deep knee bend a moment. How many ever practice this and completely straighten the knees when coming to the erect position. The knees are invariably bent. You should always straighten the legs in all leg motions I have explained, by locking the knees. Half the effect is lost if you do not.

Long distance runners run flat foot. If they did not, the arches of the foot would quickly become pounded to death. Shrubb, Longboat, Hayes, Kolehmainen, and Nurmi all run flat foot and none of them have remarkable leg development.

I have noticed the German troops on parade, marching with their famous goose-step action. They actually walk with a locked knee, but the leg development of these troops is not out of the ordinary. Neither are the legs of the crack British troops. While they do not march in goose-step formation, yet, when marking time, at attention, and when marching, the knee is stiffened to straighten out the leg. Even the vast numbers of Swedish gymnasts who practice the gymnastic march secure no unusual leg development from that special walk. This march is fine for the calves, but more weight than the bodyweight is required to give these muscles the necessary resistance.

Years ago I was quite friendly with the famous Swiss athlete, John Lemm, who at that time was the world's greatest wrestler. He had wonderful legs, and he was the first to explain to me this difference. His occupation was divided between athletics and that of an Alpine guide.

226

Ordinary walking becomes too habitual to ever provide material leg size. If it was not so, then we would find professional walkers and long distance runners with legs the equal of the mountaineer and sprinter.

A little mental deduction will prove how illogical such an idea is. The muscles of the body are given to us to adequately take care of all our physical movements. This is the reason why the muscles do not grow from merely carrying the bodyweight. Try to build a big thigh or biceps with a pair of two-pound dumbbells. It can't be done. You must give the muscles the necessary amount of resistance and they grow, in order to be more capable of handling the greater weight. In other words, the greater the material resistance, the greater the muscular growth.

Before I had been properly informed of the difference between employing the calf muscles and the effect of the Achilles tendon in walking, climbing, sprinting and distance running, I was always mentally wrestling with the problem of why the red Indian, who could carry freight on the tump line over portages and mountain trail in the wilderness, never showed any exceptional leg development. These men are capable of handling heavy loads and shamble along all day in that peculiar hodge-podge gait, that literally eats up distance. After receiving enlightenment I noticed that the Indian trailed flat foot under the tump line, and never appeared to straighten his knee. I have done a lot of road work for improving the wind in my time, but any improvement I got for my legs was obtained from the intensive training of home exercise.

CHAPTER XVII
WHERE IS THE SCIENCE OF LIFTING WEIGHTS?

If we wish to be successful in any of our undertakings we are obliged to study the scientific side of the subject, no matter what it may be. No business man overlooks this important question, which is true of selling cloth or erecting bridges. The man who pitches the ball over the plate and the salesman must each study the separate science that is involved in their respective vocations. Years ago the word science was explained as "knack" in pitching a baseball, and the salesman's tongue was termed "slick." It may still be true, if you want to put it that way, but we know that the great pitchers have all studied how to hold a ball to send the baffling curve from the box just as the successful salesman studies human psychology.

No person was ever born with the knack of doing a thing so well that it placed him in the top-notch class. There is no doubt many men have a natural ability to do one certain thing much better than others can do it, but if he is wise enough to recognize that trait, he concentrates upon the cultivation of his natural ability and becomes, to a large extent, invariably successful.

Science is recognized in sports much more readily than elsewhere, because all mechanical aid is taken away and the athlete has to resort more to his skill and physical ability to accomplish the best that is in him. Practically speaking, the skill an athlete exhibits is a practical demonstration of his scientific knowledge. As long as he receives no mechanical aid, there is no trickery in his science. Everything depends upon his skillful co-ordination of mind and body. The ability of a boxer or wrestler to outguess his opponent is as valuable as that of the crack billiard player to sense where the ball will break upon the green blaize; or of the weight- lifter who knows the leverage principles as applied to the muscles in lifting weights, and the law of gravity as it controls the actions of a weight. No other sport involves such a deep knowledge of these principles as is required by the sport of lifting weights. By the application of correct exercise, and the study of the body, and by knowing the fundamentals of the laws of resistance, any man can become more than normally efficient in this sport. This is not the case in sprinting or jumping. A man first has to have considerable natural ability in these directions, and his training is done more with an eye to intensify his speed and nervous force, rather than to build up his body. Experience has taught that weight-lifting as a sport is a builder, and speed racing takes such an expenditure of force that the racer does not recuperate the spent energies as quickly as is done in weight lifting, which is the main reason why a weight-lifter can continue to practice and stay at the top in his sport, while six generations of sprinters come and go.

One time I was sitting eating with a friend in a restaurant when he drew my attention to two men who were paying their checks. He explained that both these men drew a large salary for their technical knowledge, that enabled them to tell how much resistance it took to bend any size of iron or steel a fraction of an inch. These men understood the law of resistance in a different sense from that in which we shall use it, but the end to be gained is the same. They understood resistance as applied on material inert force, while the weight lifter must understand its application to the physical living force. The muscles of the body resist like the structural column of a building, the only difference being the latter resists by its support and the former by its active opposition. Both are a matter of strength.

Many people, unfortunately, do not comprehend the full significance of science in lifting heavy weights. They say skill in weight lifting is nothing but a trick, although at the same time they concede that the use of skill in such sports as baseball or tennis is legitimate. Still, I realize that we have a habit of using the word "trick," and do not always mean it in the sense of a fake. It is mostly used to explain the knack or science, of a sport we do not fully understand. It is not given for us to be good at everything, therefore, we are not able to fully understand the science of everything, but we can at least be appreciative.

The sport of lifting calls for more science than any other sport, simply because there are many more phases or sides to it. There are numerous lifts, each of which calls for a varied technique. I have heard it suggested that if any lifter is the strongest man in the world, he ought to hold the highest mark in every lift. How utterly out of reason such a belief is shown by other sports that do not embrace a third of the technicalities employed in weight lifting. You never heard of a football star, who could play every position on the team, well enough to be All-American at them all, or with occasional exceptions, of a pitcher who could hit decently, let alone play any position on the diamond as well as he could pitch. Condensing it further, where is the stroke in an eight who can pull an oar in any part of the boat as well as in his appointed place; or a sprinter, who held every record over the short distances, let alone all the track records. Then, we could not logically expect any more of a weight lifter. I believe it is generally understood that in order to become thoroughly efficient in this sport the athlete's body must be built to a well-balanced scale. This being understood, I will pass on to talk about the scientific side of the sport. As I have previously given you to understand, the common foe of the weight lifter is gravity. The lifter has to learn to overcome this law as much as possible without resorting to artificial aid. In the same sense, the catcher behind the bat has to know how to catch the fast ball in order to minimize its force. In the sport of weight lifting this is called "timing." Of course, every sport has its timing, but where lifting a weight is the issue, a greater mathematical deduction is required. In all such lifts, as the one and two hands snatch, the swing, and clean and jerks, speed is the greatest factor to oppose gravity. Take it this way. Suppose you were pulling a weight to the shoulders in one clean movement; if the weight was fairly light for you it would be pulled to the chest as you came erect, but if the weight was very heavy, the movement would stop as it reached midway between the knee and the waist. Now, if you knew the principles of muscular leverage you would know that the arms play a rather unimportant part in pulling a weight to the chest in one movement. It is the strength of the back and the thighs that supplies the largest quota of power. If the proper amount of physical vigor is supplied, the weight will be snapped off the floor to a certain height, but, as the back and legs straighten, their power of propulsion is lessened until it becomes neutral. When you have determined the point where your pulling-in strength diminishes, it is time for you to call into action the co-ordinating factors of physical speed, which is nervous energy combined with strength. Like a flash you must release the contraction of the thigh muscles and make a deep knee bend as your arms travel under the weight, with elbows pointed forward. Practically speaking, your thigh muscles should collapse under the weight. The ordinary person may think this is easy, but it is not. Increditable speed is called for to allow your body to descend low enough so you can get under the weight. Ordinarily, the legs seem unable to move under such pressure; they act like sticks that cannot be bent. Only quick thinking and rapid co-ordination, with the operation of the right muscles, succeed here.

Here is exactly what happens. As you exert your strength to pull the weight off the floor, the greatest amount of force is expended as the back begins to straighten. This effort is only sufficient to carry the weight to a certain height, then it begins to lose its momentum, and gravity begins to assert its forces and the weight begins to descend. Really two things happen. As the back loses its leverage the weight loses its carrying force. As these two forces lose out you have to do something else to defeat the material resistance.

Wait! Let us consider it this way. Take a stone and throw it straight up in the air, and watch it closely. At first, the stone will start skywards with a rush, gradually it will slow up, then for a fraction of time it will seem to hang suspended in the air before it descends. As it comes down, how do you catch it? You don't cup the hands and stand stiff legged and receive the whole shock of the falling stone. Not at all, you give at the knees a little to absorb the shock. This being true, what happens as you throw up a heavier stone. Why! it does not soar as high, and its descent is more rapid, and you find you have to give more at the knees to enable you to sustain the greater shock. Now that is just what happens with a weight as it is pulled in to the chest, and so you must dip as you receive the weight at the shoulders. The only difference being that at the point where the weight loses its flight, and becomes suspended in the air like the stone, for that brief fraction of time, you dip and get under the weight before it gathers too much speed in its descent, and the dip helps to take away the concussion of the weight when received.

The place where the observant lifter looks for this to happen is about the line of the stomach. A fast worker can catch the weight successfully if it travels no further than the line of the navel. Anyhow, as the weight becomes heavier, the pulling height lessens, but a skillful athlete learns to time where a weight is likely to lose momentum in its various transitory stages. Also, an intuitive sense is developed that signals as a weight is dying. This is better understood as the co-ordination between mind and matter.

Every athlete develops this sense, which is often spoken of as "outguessing."

A big controlling factor in opposing gravity is the height of the person. This is a circumstance which at first thought does not seem true. It is generally believed that a short person is better at this game than a tall person, particularly at pulling in the weight to the chest, because, as the average person says, "he is closer to the weight." Well, there is such a thing as being too close to the weight. If you do not believe it, just try raising some object with a stick as a lever. Contrary to common belief, the tall man is naturally better fitted than the short man to succeed at a clean pull-in. He can secure a longer back leverage and a deeper knee bend, all of which enables him to bend over further. His pull-in is more powerful. This is proven by the fact that most of the best clean records are performed by men over the average height. Of course, Cadine and Rigoulot are not what we would call tall, but they are over the average height, and when we speak of a short person, it is in the sense that he is less than the average height. Yet, there must be a reason why these men are so good, and also Moerke, who is very short. The reason is a different application of principle.

Somehow I have come to this point of the discussion a little earlier in this chapter than I expected, so while I am here I want to have sink in your mind one very particular lesson. Many young lifters have written to me asking how to do a certain lift. I explained to them the best I possibly could in a letter, but with always an emphasis on the words that they must consider the possible necessity of a variation of the regular principle. If I have a pupil before me I can put him right on the spot, as my experience enables me to see immediately his peculiarity, as occasioned by his physical construction. Seldom do we see a man actually imitate another in style. The change of a foot, or some other little thing, on which the success of the lifter has depended, makes the slight variation. Emphatically, I say for every would-be lifter, to accept the general principle by all means, but apply your intelligence to locate your point of control. Educate yourself to the principles, but employ your intelligence. It is the intelligence of generations that has accumulated the science of weight lifting, and by its genius created the formula of education, which makes it possible to grasp the fundamentals, once properly learned. But intelligent application will be always required. It is this that has made such remarkable clean lifters of the two Frenchmen and the German Moerke. They have combined certain laws to overcome resistance. Quite a number of years ago the Swedish lifters used a method which became known as the "Swedish Hang." The lifter would take the weight off the floor rather slowly, and when the weight was almost the height of the knees, they threw their weight backwards with all their power and dipped under the weight. This caused the weight to travel towards them in a slanting line rather than in a perpendicular line. This is a law I have always taught, in just the words the term conveys. The weight must be pulled "in," not "up," but "in towards." While the natural foe of the lifter is gravity, his natural fault is lack of centralization. If you pull a weight "up," by the time it is where it should be it is hanging out in front of the body an inch or two more than it should be. The lifter has to step forward to meet it. If the weight is pulled "in" you are in the right place to receive it, with all the physical forces of the body marshaled to distribute their powers more forcibly where they may be required.

Steinborn does the same thing, and so does Klein. If you saw them lift you would imagine that they were not going to succeed, then, like lightning, they "pull" the weight "in" and are under it. Tall men can use this method to as good an advantage as the short man. The only difference is he does not have to, but the short man's short back purchase makes the method more adaptable for him. It is this same reason why, when making a two arm snatch lift plates of a low height are preferred. Here is one lift where the shorter man does excel, not so much for any leverage advantage he may have, as because he has more concentrated energy than the taller man. His nervous force is distributed over a less area and in the snatch his limitation of pulling is decreased, as compared with the clean lift to the shoulders. But in this lift, centralization is the key to success. Again I must admonish all lifters that the weight must be snatched to arms' length in an oblique line overhead, not a perpendicular line. Just stand over an imaginary weight and snatch slowly with your hands, then stop at a line level with your eyes, and if you place a stick upright with the floor and your hands you will find you are away off center. We say that the weight must be snatched to arms' length "overhead." Then see that it goes over the head so your forces can co-ordinate, and not expect a few isolated muscles to do the impossible. Pull the weight towards you and snap under it. Speed and strength are intensified more in this lift than in any other one lift. No crack representative of any other sport moves his forces as swiftly as the two arm snatcher. The greater the amount of weight he is able to snatch the faster he must be.

This reminds me of an amusing incident of which I was a spectator. Some young baseball players were belittling the merits of a rival pitcher, and in giving advice to the Babe Ruth of the team, they informed him all he had to do was to get a "line on the ball" and he would make a piker of the rival pitcher. Sounds good to a novice, but getting a line on that ball was like a novice getting a line on gravity. It takes some doing, and at first you are apt to be made the piker. Incidentally, people with that kind of advice never seem to be able to practice what they preach. You will find it takes a great deal of mind co-ordination to control the right muscles in the right place, but, like shooting at a bull's-eye with a rifle, practice makes perfect.

Jerking a weight with two arms to arms' length overhead is not fraught with as much difficulty as is the case in taking a weight off the floor to the chest in one movement. This is proven by the clean and jerk records, which are lower than the records in the two hands continental style, which allows the lifter to use two or more movements in getting the weight to the chest. Just the same, gravity appears to react more quickly in the second stage of this lift than from the ground to shoulders. Really it does not; it is the difference in the motive power employed, which is explained by the fact that a heavy weight can be lowered more slowly to the ground than it can be lowered from arms' length overhead down to the shoulders. This apparently contradictory fact may confuse your mind, as you remember I told you it was easier to succeed in lifting from the shoulders than from the ground. It is the sustaining force that is reversed. Suppose you jerk a weight aloft, and it only goes part of the way up. You find that with a combined leg dip and arm pressure against the weight you are able to finish the lift. Your sustaining powers are directed entirely beneath the weight. From the ground to the shoulders the sustaining force is above the weight, which enables you to lower a greater weight slowly to the floor than you can raise to the chest. But, when jerking overhead, you will find many athletes who jerk the weight to arms' length and fail to hold it. When such is the case, it is caused through lack of centralization, and failing to dip under the weight at the right time. You see, there is what lifters call a "dying point" in all lifts; this is the place, as explained before, where the weight loses its momentum, and the muscular leverage diminishes. In jerking a weight overhead the dying point is between the crown of the head and about three inches past it. In this space leverage is neutralized and physical resistance is lessened. In order to offset this you must dip under the weight and press against it, which enables a lifter to straighten his arms under the weight in order to complete the lift. A speedy lifter will snap the weight on to its journey, and, like a flash get underneath, but if this is not backed up by a certain amount of sustaining power the reaction takes place like a flash and the weight is speedily back where it started. We know that men like Rigoulot, Cadine, Strassberger and Steinborn are fast men, with more than the usual amount of sustaining force, and men like Swoboda, Alzin, Giroux and Moerke have greater sustaining power rather than greater speed, which makes it possible for them to slow up gravitation, just enough to allow them to finish the lift. Gorner, Steinbach and Neuhaus have both these powers, but in a greater degree than that is possessed by the other lifters. In each case these men named have centralization, leverage and the laws of resistance figured out to a fraction. They know the value of mathematical deduction, and always apply arithmetic in lifting. It is as necessary for the lifter to understand how a weight decreases in its transitory flight as the poundage becomes increased, as it is necessary for the deep sea diver to understand why he cannot dive below a certain depth. In each case it is the resistance per square inch, and each can be figured out almost exactly. At one time this was a great hobby of mine, and I have often proven in demonstration just where the dying, or sticking place was in each lift, and have shown how it was possible to overcome it with one of the many co-ordinating factors, such as speed, strength, leverage and sustaining force. Some men who jerk overhead are satisfied if they can jerk the weight to the height of the crown of the head. These men are capable of great sustaining force and can resist to an extraordinary degree. But the theory that a man who can jerk a weight a less height than other and succeed "is more tricky," as some say, or less strong, is ridiculous. He is the man who is terrifically strong. He has to be.

I once took part in a demonstrative debate on this point. My opponent said, "Look how high that man can jerk the weight (referring to a well-known Polish lightweight, now in the country), which is a record for his class." I agreed, but I replied that he does not hold the weight and such a lift is not considered. Now, I argued, let us prove him according to lifting rules, which say he must hold the weight for a count of one, two, and stand erect under it. Right away the lifter dropped from 250 pounds to 225 pounds, which is a poundage that can be surpassed by many lightweight lifters. The moral is this: The Polish lifter had no sustaining force, and to prove my assertion I told my lifter to lift as the Pole did, and he went away up in his poundage to about three hundred pounds. However, that is not lifting. Rarely do we come across men with such great sustaining force; but when we do, we find they are always men who have a complete mastery over the leverage principles of their muscles, and know just when and where to apply them, much as a motorist knows when to shift his gears when climbing a steep hill.

Take the one hand swing for another example of applied science. Here is a lift that calls for many changes and a lightning coordination of all the forces, that result in making it bewildering to the novice. In this country, we swing with a straight arm throughout the lift, as is practiced in Europe. The British have a style of their own, of which I do not approve, as a genuine swing. They used to swing in the accepted style. However, in this lift the weight is carried to a point where there is absolutely no physical control over it—when the weight is traveling at right angles to the body. We all know that no lifter could possibly hold the weight out that is swung at right angle by sheer strength. It must be carried past that point by the sheer force of the sweep taken off the floor. Most lifters only get a quarter swing out of their sweep, because they do not co- ordinate. Now an intelligent survey will show you that for about two-thirds of the distance the weight is traveling away from the body, that is, if you swing right. But to be successful in this lift, every inch of the way, the weight must be controlled. A quarter swing is the cause of lack of centralization, and uncontrolled gravity. The real swing lifter sends the bell sweeping through the air in a half circle, which keeps the weight traveling towards him, as it passes the dead line. In order to do this he must pull backwards with his body as he comes erect, which turns the arc of the weight from a quarter circle to a half circle, and thus carries it past the dead line, traveling towards him from the half-way point. A lot more has still to be done, for the flight of the weight may not be high enough, which would cause his arms to bend. As soon as the weight is felt to pass the turning point, he thrusts with the straight arm against the weight and steps forward to meet it with the lifting foot advanced. Thus a connection is made by meeting the weight as it travels towards the lifter, offsetting gravity, and centralizing the forces. Stepping forward takes the place of a dip and lowers the body under the weight.

This thrust may seem vague to the beginner, so let us find an ordinary circumstance with which you will be familiar, to illustrate visually what is meant. At some time you have seen a big door, or some similar object, blown over by the wind, and as you rush to save it from the fall you thrust against it with the hands. However, you may recollect that natural instinct caused you to employ a straight arm, and with your weight thrown behind the arm thrust the heavy door was propped back in place. If your arms bent at the elbow the door beat you, and the arms became like broken props. Now, that is just what happens in a swing. If the arm is bent, no leverage is registered; if it is straight, it becomes a rigid prop of advantage, and the bodily strength springing forward its reserve, completes the whole show. It is a fast lift, and calls for quicker thinking, faster action, and more vigorous strength in one combined effort than any other lift. Greater skill is required, and the man who excels on this lift with a good poundage hung up as his record is apt to be a good, all-round lifter.

The bent press is always considered a very skillful lift, and, incidentally, is a lift that always brings up a controversy. Some argue that it is purely a case of knack, without any expenditure of strength required. Now, if it is solely a balancing feat, why cannot everybody succeed with it? However, when I hear a person talk that way I am quite sure I am listening to one who is not good in the bent press. I think it is a very useful lift, due to the value attached to it in teaching a lifter to know how to control a heavy weight. It gets the body accustomed to overcome greater resistance. It is barred from use in national, or world's competition, largely because it is not a universal lift. Anyhow, let us study it for the value of what it teaches us. We will concede the point to the argumentative chorus, and say it is a balancing feat, but to suggest that no strength is required is a theory exploded at the very beginning of the lift. The weight must be taken to the shoulder first. Now show me the average strong man who can toy with two hundred pounds in one hand at the shoulder, even if someone is helping him to the shoulder. Why! he is anchored. He cannot move with it. Then what on earth would he do with it at arms' length? No matter how well centralized a lifter is, or how he balances a weight, the skill applied cannot lessen the weight of the object. Two hundred pounds will always register two hundred pounds of pressure, and the longer the weight is held the greater the depression that is registered. It takes power to hold the weight, even if it is balanced in such a position as to make its passage from the shoulder to arms' length easy, and the lifter must stand erect under it. Even if we consider it a balancing feat, strength is an absolute necessity. Somehow, it savors a little of the story of Pat and Mike. A big bale fell on Pat and pinned him to the ground. He roared for Mike to pull it off, but Mike informed him if he got under the bale he ought to be able to get from under it. No great strength was required to get under the bale, but it certainly was required to get from under it. At one time, and that is not a great while ago, all that was required to call a bent press a lift was to bend under until the straight arm was secured. Later, when the sport became organized, the lifter was obliged to stand erect with the weight at arms' length. Then what became of all those bent press agents? They simply could not make the grade. A centralized poise is the main issue in this lift, but when a man begins to handle two hundred and fifty pounds and over and do the lift correctly, you will always find that he has enough power to do other lifts with a meritorious poundage, as well as the bent press.

In most sports, all an athlete has to handle is his weight; the lifter has to have the power to handle his own weight and another weight, that invariably exceeds his own bodyweight considerably. He is the one athlete who must possess dynamic force. It often takes years to become an accomplished all-round lifter. The brilliant performer of today did not succeed in a few months. It took time and study. The science of the sport was not all compiled in a day, either, nor by any one man. It has taken generations of lifters to cultivate the skill that the sport now embraces. The skill of boxing is made up of blocks, blows and stops, plus speed and stamina. The skill of wrestling consists of locks, blocks, breaks, and bars, plus speed and stamina. Every sport has its special line of science, but the science of weight lifting always resolves itself upon the amount of knowledge possessed by the lifter on the muscular principles of leverage, mathematical deduction of timing a weight, the sustaining power of the combined physical forces, co-ordination between mind and body, plus speed, strength, stamina and a well-balanced muscular body. The greater success of the present time heavy weight lifter in handling heavy weights over the strong man of a generation ago is the result of better teamwork within himself, that has brought his co-ordination to a higher plane of perfection.

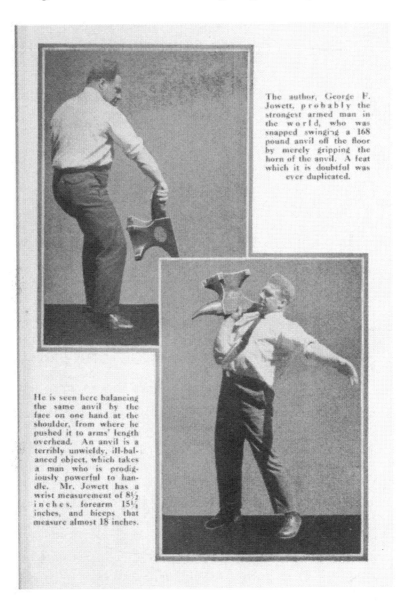

The author, George F. Jowett, probably the strongest armed man in the world, who was snapped swinging a 168 pound anvil off the floor by merely gripping the horn of the anvil. A feat which it is doubtful was ever duplicated.

He is seen here balancing the same anvil by the face on one hand at the shoulder, from where he pushed it to arms' length overhead. An anvil is a terribly unwieldy, ill-balanced object, which takes a man who is prodigiously powerful to handle. Mr. Jowett has a wrist measurement of 8½ inches, forearm 15½ inches, and biceps that measure almost 18 inches.

Arthur Pell, a famous English strong man who hails from the same quarter as Louis Hardt, Thomas Inch, Ed Aston, "Teddy" Mack, and E. C. Smith, all men famous for their might and muscle.

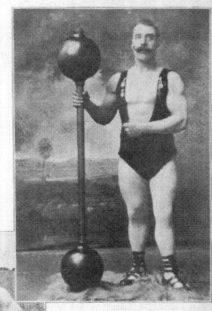

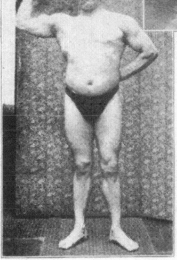

Louis Vasseur, the great French veteran, who many years ago showed the great possibilities in the quick lifts. He has snatched with one hand over 220 pounds. Although well on in his fifties, he is still a dangerous challenger for the world's proudest title.

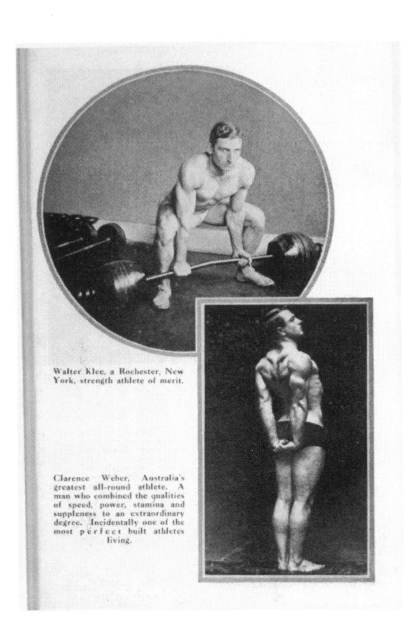

Walter Klee, a Rochester, New York, strength athlete of merit.

Clarence Weber, Australia's greatest all-round athlete. A man who combined the qualities of speed, power, stamina and suppleness to an extraordinary degree. Incidentally one of the most perfect built athletes living.

Ottley R. Coulter, Union-
town, Pennsylvania, a star
athlete who has been
a monument of force in
furthering the cause of
physical training. He was
the world's lightweight
back and harness lifting
champion, and ran second
place to Warren Lincoln
Travis in the Brooklyn
contest of 1918 for the
Police Gazette Belt.

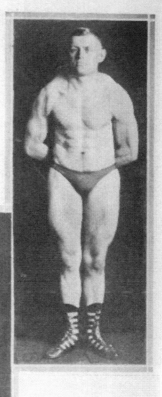

Robert Jennings, a power-
ful wrestler whose ability
to hold out weights in the
crucifix position is amazing. At 147 pounds body-
weight, he has held out
75 pounds in each hand.

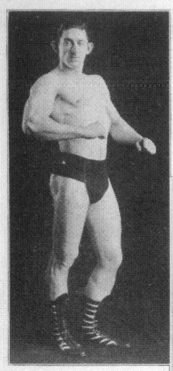

Albert Manger, of Baltimore, one of the finest present day younger generation of American strong men. His fine physique and splendid feats of strength and rapid rise from a physical state that was below average, has made him the center of attraction in strength sport.

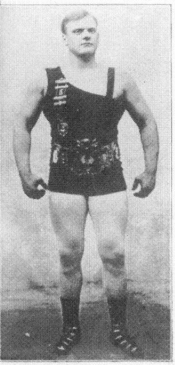

Warren Lincoln Travis, of New York, who stands supreme as the world's greatest back and harness lifter. His phenomenal two finger lift of 860 pounds was only eclipsed by the astounding performance with which he celebrated his fiftieth birthday. He is a native son, of which America is proud.

Alfred Alzin, of Marseilles, stands six feet three inches and weighs 326 pounds. His terrific strength runs him close to Gorner. Recently on ten lifts he accumulated a total that swamped the totals of Rigoulot and Cadine, on the same lifts.

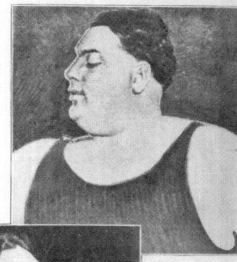

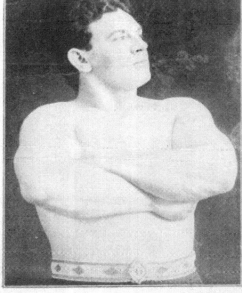

Hector De Carrie, of Montreal, who succeeded Cyr to the title. A strength athlete with a vivid career who could always do 275 pounds with two dumb-bells and claims to have bent pressed around 325 pounds.

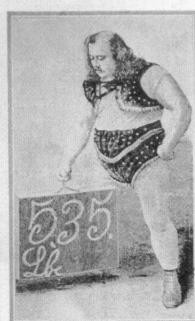

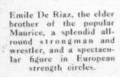

The mighty Louis Cyr, for years considered the "Daddy of 'em all." This picture was taken from an old drawing made when he was in his heyday of glory, illustrating his one finger lift of 535 pounds.

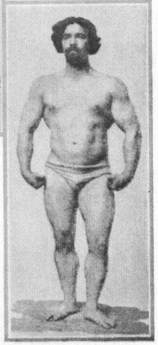

Emile De Riaz, the elder brother of the popular Maurice, a splendid all-round strongman and wrestler, and a spectacular figure in European strength circles.

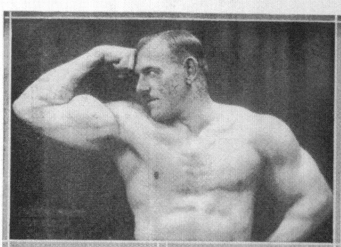

The mighty Gorner displaying his lusty 18½ inch biceps, 16 inch forearm, 20 inch neck and 52½ inch chest. Truly a pillar of power.

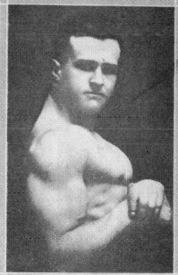

The magnificent development of the breast muscles and biceps are splendidly depicted in this pleasing pose of Earle E. Liederman.

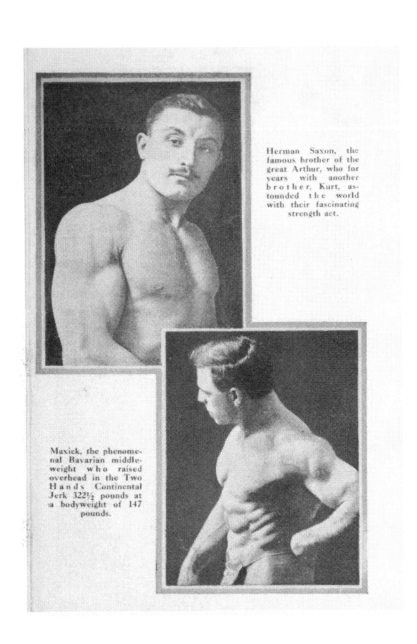

Herman Saxon, the famous brother of the great Arthur, who for years with another brother, Kurt, astounded the world with their fascinating strength act.

Maxick, the phenomenal Bavarian middleweight who raised overhead in the Two Hands Continental Jerk 322½ pounds at a bodyweight of 147 pounds.

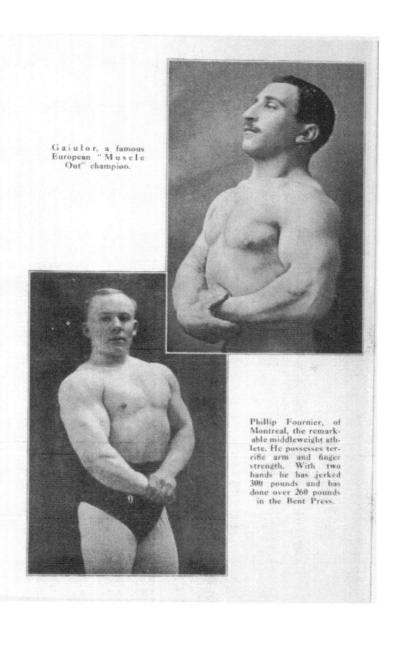

Gaiulor, a famous
European "Muscle
Out" champion.

Phillip Fournier, of
Montreal, the remark-
able middleweight ath-
lete. He possesses ter-
rific arm and finger
strength. With two
hands he has jerked
300 pounds and has
done over 260 pounds
in the Bent Press.

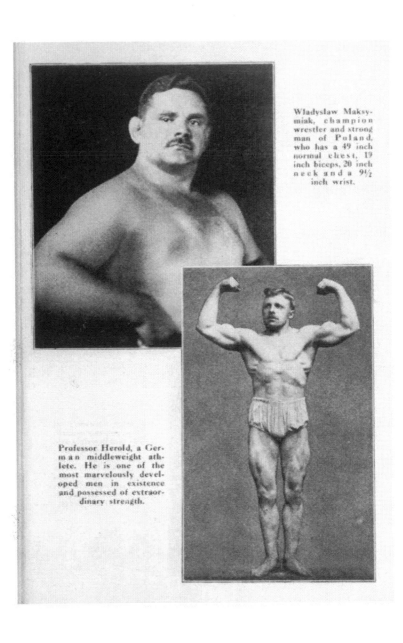

Wladyslaw Maksy-
miak, champion
wrestler and strong
man of Poland,
who has a 49 inch
normal chest, 19
inch biceps, 20 inch
neck and a 9½
inch wrist.

Professor Herold, a Ger-
m a n middleweight ath-
lete. He is one of the
most marvelously devel-
oped men in existence
and possessed of extraor-
dinary strength.

Launceston Elliott, London, was considered the most perfectly built man of his day. He stood six feet one and a half inches, weighing 244 pounds, chest 50 inches normal, biceps 18½ inches, forearm 15½ inches, hips 42 inches, thigh 31 inches, calf 18½ inches, neck 18¾ inches, waist 36 inches. Won world's amateur weight lifting championship at Athens 1896. Started handling weights at the age of fifteen years.

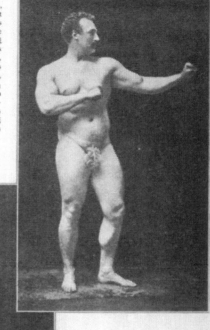

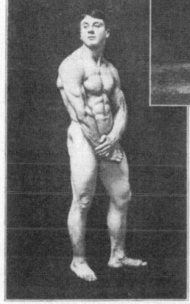

Monte Saldo, London. Another English strength athlete with exceptional muscular development. He was the first man to ever swing more than his own bodyweight with one hand, swinging over 150 pounds at a bodyweight of 147 pounds.

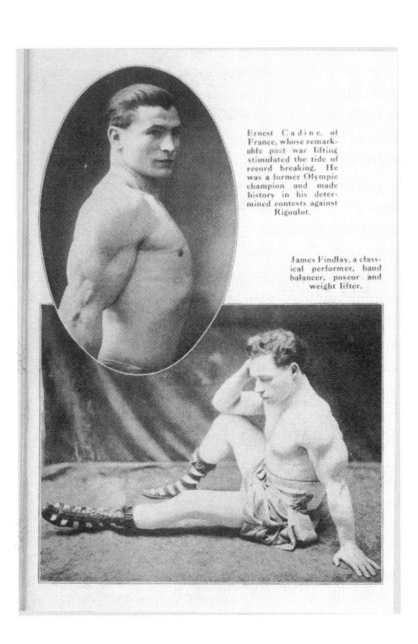

Ernest Cadine, of France, whose remarkable post war lifting stimulated the tide of record breaking. He was a former Olympic champion and made history in his determined contests against Rigoulot.

James Findlay, a classical performer, hand balancer, poseur and weight lifter.

This photo was snapped of Carl Moerke as he concluded a Two Hands Continental Jerk of 375 pounds.

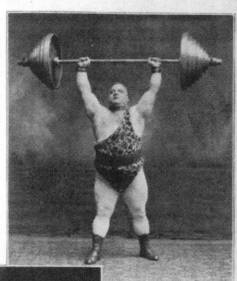

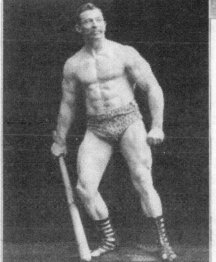

No man has ever so clearly depicted the great possibilities of manly beauty as Staff Serj. Moss. There is more to admire in his bodily contour than that of a woman. He ranks with such other symmetrical luminaries as MacMahon and Pandour.

255

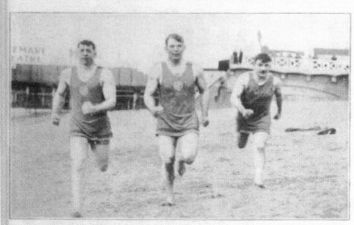

Noah Young, weight lifting champion, Frank Gotch world's wrestling champion, and Dan McCloud, middleweight wrestling star, dashing for the beach at Los Angeles, California.

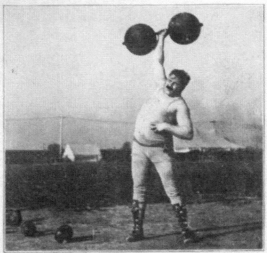

Fred Winters, the first American Olympic weight lifting champion.

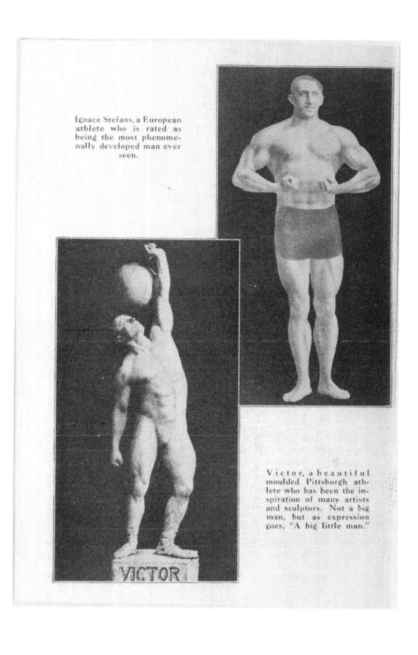

Ignace Stefans, a European athlete who is rated as being the most phenomenally developed man ever seen.

Victor, a beautiful moulded Pittsburgh athlete who has been the inspiration of many artists and sculptors. Not a big man, but as expression goes, "A big little man."

CHAPTER XVIII
BUILDING A SHAPELY ARM

When Sandow started a wave of enthusiasm for physical training throughout the world by the demonstration of his beautiful physique, his admiring followers were entranced with the beauty of his perfectly built arm. It was a sight that started many off on the quest for a similar arm, but very few obtained one like Sandow. At the time his biceps' measurement was only a little over sixteen inches; it had the appearance of being eighteen inches. Sandow was fortunate by nature in having clean-cut joints. This, combined with the shapeliness of his arm, made his biceps appear very massive. He also possessed a thin skin, which allowed the muscular separation to stand out with a very pronounced distinction. I have heard some people remark that the public had never seen such beautifully shaped muscles before the advent of Eugene Sandow, but I would not say that, for I know that there were other beautiful specimen of physical manhood at that time, but they lacked that something, whether it was showmanship or popularity, that put Sandow over. This, no doubt, was the reason why they were overlooked while the world was lionizing the famous inspiration of Audrey Hunt. However, it seems that every young man's idea of being strong and well built consists of being able to show a big biceps. Well, I certainly like to see a well shaped arm, pro- viding it is balanced and symmetrical, but I dislike a big biceps that does not show forearm and triceps development to balance it. Performers on Roman rings generally have large biceps. I knew one young man who only weighed one hundred and twenty pounds and he had a sixteen inch biceps and stood less than five feet three inches in height. He was a marvel on the rings; but a sixteen inch biceps on a man so light in weight and so short is out of all proportion.

His upper arm looked larger than his thighs. Chinning fiends get the same development. A fine looking young chap came to me one time and told me he would like to be a good hand balancer, but he was not able to straighten out his arm to make a hand stand. I asked him what he was best at, and right away he began telling me how many times he could chin himself. He rolled up his sleeve and showed me a mighty fine biceps, but he had practically no triceps worth speaking about. I told him if he would devote as much time daily to his triceps development for the next four weeks as he had to his biceps work, and leave out the chinning, he would then have what I termed a real arm and, besides, become capable of doing hand stands. It did not take him four weeks. Three weeks later he came to see me and you should have seen those triceps. The arm was beautiful.

Just notice any mechanic who is using a hammer all day. You will see a nice looking arm, but notice how his arm is bent at the elbow. With so much flexion of the arm the biceps have become shortened, and to straighten the arm out is almost painful in some cases. If you do any amount of heavy shoveling the same condition will come about. No man can become a successful weight lifter, or hand balancer—understander as well as top mounter—unless he displays a perfectly balanced arm. Therein lies the real secret of arm strength, and if there should be any disproportion it should favor the triceps and not the biceps. The triceps is an extensor muscle, and the biceps is a flexor.

I have often advised arm builders to practice chinning, and I do yet, but the trouble with the chinning fiend is that he never fully straightens his arm out; and the more tired he becomes the less he straightens his arm. That is where he is wrong. If he straightened his arm out completely, as he lowers his weight, the biceps would receive full extension as well as contraction. The supinator longus will straighten the arm more than the triceps will in chinning, but the triceps get a little action.

Some men find their bodyweight too heavy to handle in chinning, especially when they are around two hundred pounds, and have had no previous experience. But by following the advice I will give here they will not be deprived of the benefits of chinning. Tie two lengths of rope on a bar-bell and pass these ropes through a couple of pulleys placed in the ceiling, or throw the ropes over a horizontal bar. Take the two loose ends and tie a stick in them for a handle, then pull on the stick with both hands. You will be obliged to experiment a little before you know to what weight to load the bar bell in order to pull up. Pull on the handle bar until it is at your chest, just the same as if you were chinning yourself on a bar. This method will satisfactorily answer the purpose, and give you a good workout.

Curling dumb-bells and bar bells is another standby of the big biceps boys. I often watch them, but I seldom see them carry out the real idea of a one or two arm curl. Maybe the first two or three curls are fair, but soon I begin to see them lean forward and then the curl becomes shortened from not lowering the weight enough. It might interest you to know that the two-arm curl is a stunt which a weight lifter likes to see his opponent try before a match. Sometimes he will even try to get him to warm up with it. If he succeeds in doing this he will try to start the contest off with a two hands snatch, and force the pace. The other lifter, knowing his possibilities, will start near his limit. To his amazement he finds that while the weight is snatched, yet it comes down before he can lock his arms. Generally he becomes rash and uses up his three attempts with the same weight or a heavier one, and fails each time. This is the penalty of curling before the contest. His biceps become shortened just enough so that it prevented him from locking his arms, and the match is lost.

When an exerciser gets to about fifty per cent, of his body- weight in the two-arm curl I like to see him make a change. Not because this amount of weight will shorten his biceps, but because the two-arm curl brings about a depression of the diaphragm, which has a similar effect to that produced by the two-arm Pull Over when using too much weight. In the place of the bar-bell curl I advise curling with a pair of kettle-weights. You may ask yourself, "What is the difference?" A great deal. In the first place a greater extension of the biceps is given, and a longer pull is secured, which develops the muscle in a more capable manner, and makes it strong every part of the way.

Sometime or other you may have tried to do a feat that a friend of yours did, or perhaps you saw a stunt at the vaudeville theatre you wanted to duplicate and you failed. Do you ever remember remarking to your friend how you almost got it, but at a certain angle your muscles did not have just the right power? That is because your muscles lacked the full power in their pull. The cables of connection lacked the power, or else the contraction of the muscle fibers was not sufficient at that one point for the appointed task. Perhaps by now you will see the value of my constant urge to always give the muscles their full play when exercising them. What is the use of half educating them ? Nothing is right unless it is done correctly. Getting back to where I left off on the curl, let me say that the divided action prevents any diaphragm compression. Curl the kettle weights simultaneously and curl them separately. Use dumb-bells also, curl them endways for a change; bend over from the waist and while in that position curl one of them to the shoulder without standing erect. Keep the other hand on the knee for a support. If you raise a pair of fairly heavy dumb-bells overhead, and then slowly lower them by bending the arm at the elbow, until the upper arm is level with the shoulder, you will find the action of the biceps again different. Develop your muscles from every conceivable angle. Then their quality becomes better in construction, as well as in action.

The biceps has a double head, as its name implies. They also have a double insertion, and the two bellies unite into one tendon that is attached deeply in the hollow of the elbow joint. The action of the muscle is described as being of the shoulder and humeroradial and radial ulnar joint, and altogether it is an extremely variable muscle. It has been known to have possessed a third head of origin, and rated at ten per cent., which is the reason why some people naturally seem to have larger and better formed biceps than others. Some diligent arm builders have been very puzzled over the fact that while their biceps registered only a slow gain in size, their biceps strength has increased out of all proportion to its gain in size. Invariably they attribute this to the possession of a longer humerus bone than the average. That is the bone of the upper arm. This condition is common among tall people, although once in a while I do come across a short person with a longer upper arm than usual. However, that makes no difference, but it is an actual fact that a person who has a longer humerus will have a stronger arm all-round. This is not due to having more muscular tissue over a greater space. The source of power is found in the longer attachment, which is seated further up on the bone of the forearm. This gives the biceps a greater leverage, and makes flexion of the forearm upon the upper arm easier. The individual thus constructed is capable of pulling a weight off the floor to the shoulder more easily, and also of raising a weight to arms' length in a jerk movement more readily.

The biceps has a peculiar method of shaping itself as it grows larger. In some cases it shapes itself like a ball, showing a groove where both heads separate. On the other hand, some biceps just become a mass of muscle that completely fills up the entire space on the upper arm. The tissue at the elbow joint will be almost as dense as it is further up the arm. This generally signifies very thick ligaments, and it is often the more powerful muscle of the two. This type of muscle is more apt to be like good rubber when relaxed, and hard when tensed. I have noticed the ball-shaped muscle is inclined to be very hard when tensed and there is not a great deal of change when relaxed; but the latter is by far the more admirable muscle from the standpoint of its beautiful shapliness. Yet, if they lack a certain amount of depth at the elbow joint, they take on a grotesque appearance. Personally, I never like to see anything abnormal in muscular development. No matter how large or small muscles may be, they can all acquire symmetry.

Otto Arco and Sam Kramer both have beautiful upper arms, and I remember that Arthur Saxon had, too. There are many who have beautifully shaped arms, but it would be useless for me to mention them, as the reader is not familiar with them. Well shaped, strong biceps are not such a rare possession. They are a gift that can be acquired by yourself. You do not have to stand by and be satisfied admiring others. However, never forget the triceps. Let us turn to these muscles now, which are actually more important and more powerful than the biceps. The next time you go to the theatre and see a hand-to-hand balancing team, just pay careful attention to the contour of the understander's arm when it is relaxed. He will have to be standing so you obtain a side view of him. Then you will see in the back of the arm a curve commencing from a little above the elbow joint which swells out as it runs up to the shoulder. This is the triceps. For a contrast, look at the upper arm of a clerk, or a salesman, or anybody who does not use the arm muscles to any great extent. In place of the curve you will see just a straight line, and probably the elbow joint will look as though it is going to stick through the skin. It might surprise you to see how weak the latter is when it comes to raising any heavy object overhead. Most of them, if they

263

had their arm cut off, would hardly miss the little good that their triceps are to them. So little are these muscles employed by the average person that their existence is very rudimentary, whereas they should be swelling and powerful. As their name implies, the triceps has three heads. They are the only muscles on the posterior part of the upper arm. Each has a lateral, a medial and a scapular origin, and becomes inserted on the forearm. In appearance, it takes the shape of a horseshoe, but one head is longer than the other, as you can easily see. The triceps is the extensor muscle of the elbow joint, but the long head also acts as an abductor of the humerus, at the shoulder joint. Because we always speak of this muscle as the one that straightens out the arm when pushing a weight overhead, it is often referred to as a pushing muscle, but as I have said before, there are no such things as pushing muscles; they all pull.

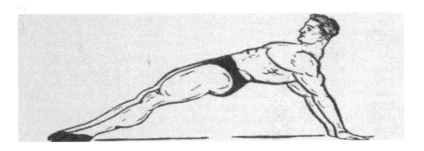

Perhaps the finest pair of triceps I ever saw are those that adorn the arm of Joseph Urlacher. They are remarkably clean-cut, and show every line of separation in their process. Unlike the majority, his triceps seem to form more deeply. I mean, that while most triceps show a great fullness closer to the shoulder, his starts to swell out from their points of insertion at the elbow. Especially the inner head. Arco has a beautifully balanced upper arm, and also Arthur Hyson, but their triceps are exceptionally well developed. Also, I can recall a slaughterman, who was employed by a butcher who had his store next door to where I once lived. I never grew weary of looking this man over. He was the most magnificent specimen of what we would call untrained manhood that I ever saw. His biceps measured seventeen inches, and he weighed around two hundred pounds. From the crown of his head to the soles of his feet he was beautifully built. I never saw him other than bare-headed, shirt throat open, and sleeves rolled up to the shoulders. Often I have seen him carry on his shoulders, from the slaughter house to the butcher shop, a distance of half a mile, a dressed beef; and incoming he had to walk up a very steep grade. When he flexed his biceps the triceps bellied out underneath in a wonderful sweep. However, no professional weight lifter ever did more heavy lifting than he. His work entailed long hours and he enjoyed using his strength in place of a block and tackle. Every muscle in his body got a workout. But those arms 1 They were a sight for the gods.

Just pushing a bar bell to arms' length is not enough, although a lot of this will develop fine triceps, but everybody does not have that amount of time to spare. Such labor is not necessary, as direct methods will give faster results that are equally as good. Here is a real good exercise. You take up your position as the illustration shows on page 231. The main thing for you to observe is that your body is kept perfectly straight. The moment it is allowed to sag at the waist the exercise becomes useless, simply because very little tricep contraction is registered. From that position, lower yourself by bending the arm, but keeping the body absolutely straight when lowering and raising. If the exercise becomes a little too easy, attach a weight to a sling and have it hanging around the forehead. This will supply you with the necessary resistance. Two more good exercises are as follows: Stand erect with a light bar bell of about twenty-five pounds hanging at arms' length, behind. From the erect position bend forwards from the waist, and at the same time, raise the bar bell as high as you can, backwards, then lower, and at the same time, straighten the body. The next exercise should give the triceps a little more kick. It always gives vigorous play to the triceps and it really has been my favorite triceps exercise. Take either a light dumb-bell, or an iron plate in your hand and stand erect with the feet spaced a suitable distance apart. From this position bend the hand back on the wrist, and do not let the palm of the hand twist sideways. Keep it facing forwards throughout the exercise; then grip the weight strongly and begin to raise the arm backwards. As you do this you will have a tendency to twist the body sideways. This you must vigorously counteract, and by so doing, a stronger pull will be given to the triceps. When the arm is at the limit of its height, pause, and then rotate the wrist and hand in a circular movement. If you do this right you will feel the triceps action very strongly. After two or three wrist rotations lower the arm and stand erect before you repeat. Work out both arms and massage the muscles after each exercise period. The severe contraction of the muscle in this exercise necessitates this procedure.

There are many movements that will give these muscles a certain amount of play, but the trouble is that the play is not sufficiently direct. All the exercises I have given are specific in their uses, as required by the various muscles. I know they will give you the very best results if you concentrate upon them as you should, and I hope you will. Unless you do you will never have a shapely arm, and when remembering about triceps exercise, don't forget that this muscle helps to swell the tape measure to sixteen inches.

CHAPTER XIX
How Specialization Destroys the Jinx of Stubborn Muscles

Some great old sage once passed the pleasant remark that "Anything worth having is worth working for, and the more desirable the object the more difficult it is of attainment." Many a young man who has started out to build a better conditioned body for himself has found the latter part of the saying to be only too true. He fully realizes that a perfect body is worth having, and he often figures that he has worked for it, but something is wrong with the work, as the progress registered is not proportionate to all his labors. Brutal as it may seem, I doubt if all have put forward the right amount of effort. Unfortunately, some believe that as long as they go through their routine, results should be obtained. Others quit too easily, and others are too impatient. They forget the amount of things that have to be taken into consideration. In the first place, thought, care and concentration are required from the moment the first movement is made in the first exercise to the very end. Impatience is the worst thing in the world, no matter where it is concerned, and the person who is afflicted in that way is as badly off as the quitter, who never gets anywhere. The old saw that "Rome was not built in a day" is still true. Some of us are not as fortunate as others, who seem to be blessed with the magic wand of Vulcan. They build up in leaps and bounds, acquiring great ability in proportion, just as some people acquire wealth easily. Still, it would not be right to expect something without working for it, and neither is it right that a person should work so hard at his exercises that he makes the time spent seem like a torture period.

Exercise is a subject that requires deep study, and calls for the guiding hand of an efficient instructor. Anybody can pick up a few exercises and by practicing them keep himself normally fit, but where the developing process starts it is a different question. A few exercises picked and practiced at random are all lost motion. The beginner does not know whether the type of exercises he has scheduled for himself are of any real value or not, but the moment an expert views his measurements he can tell just what is required, and such a man should be consulted first.

Some men make wonderful gains; their body seems to respond very readily to exercise, but in every case you will find that each of these men have applied themselves intelligently to their routine. They never for one moment viewed exercise as a fad. With them it was considered a necessity. If a man starts with a bodyweight of 125 pounds, against a height of 5' 9", it would be foolish for him to expect to build up into a 175-pound man within two or three months, or to compare his results with those of a man who started in at 165 pounds at the same height, and who in a very short time displayed a splendidly formed body with exceptional strength. The latter had less distance to go to win his goal. Therefore, the road must necessarily be a little longer and the going harder for the one who starts in underweight with an ill- shaped body and a lesser degree of manpower.

I have known a great many who within a few weeks made fine gains on one part of their body, but the rest of their body stood still. In such a case it is not necessary to become excited, as some parts of the body will always respond more quickly to exercise than others. Therefore, before any thought of specialization is considered, at least three months should be devoted to all-round exercises. Then the exercises have been given a chance to prove their value. If it is found that the biceps or the chest have not improved in proportion, the thing to do is to change the exercises, or else specialize upon the one part of the body that you most desired to improve. But this does not mean a body builder should begin to specialize immediately after putting in a few months' practice. He must give the body a chance, and as I just explained, a change of exercise should be given first. A great deal will also depend upon the actual condition in which the body may be. If the exerciser has a fairly well built body, he can start in to specialize earlier than it is advisable for the other fellow, who has a longer way to go. Just what I mean is something like this. Imagine two men, who are both five feet six inches tall, and one strips at 150 pounds and has a 15-inch neck, a 38-inch chest, 13½- inch biceps, 22-inch thigh, and 14½-inch calf, and the other fellow weighs 125 pounds stripped, with a 13½-inch neck, 35-inch chest, 12-inch upper arm, 19-inch thigh and a 13-inch calf. The former is in a much better position to commence specialized training than the other fellow, and it is always the under developed fellow who gets the most excited. Of course, we can forgive him, for we know it is only because he is very anxious to build up a body that is worthwhile. Yet, he should restrain himself and realize that his position is similar to that of one man who must walk twenty-five miles to accomplish the same object, for which the other man has to walk only twelve. It will take him a longer time. The smaller man should be content to follow a general routine for a longer time. Of course, it is quite justifiable for him to change certain exercises, but they should be included with the other regular exercises. When the time for specialization is reached, this does not mean that all other exercises for the other parts of the body must be neglected. Training on the principle of one exercising period in each forty-eight hours, the exerciser would be required to reduce the length of time devoted to the rest of the body, so greater time can be spared for the concentration of the part of the body that is below par. Training is required every night or day, from this time on, and I might say that it is a better method to select two or three parts of the body for specialization at the same time, but with first consideration given to the one part specially desired. Let us suppose that the chest is going to be our chief object, and we find that the biceps of the thigh are not developed to balance the general development of the thigh, and that the calf can also stand some extra attention. We find that we have three exercises for the chest that are calculated to give the results, so we concentrate on these; but do not get the idea in your head that the way to go after real chest improvement is to go the limit on each exercise, or that these three have to be practiced in rotation. The reason I selected two other parts of the body to work in conjunction with the chest was to offset that idea, because there is a right and wrong way to practice special training.

It is wrong to work on an exercise until you are tired out. Suppose you find fifteen movements with a certain weight fatigues you. Then the thing for you to do is to go no higher than twelve counts. Commencing upon a chest exercise you use enough repetitions so that they will make you just comfortably tired. The next exercise should be for the calf; thigh biceps after that; and then come back with another chest exercise. Then, just as before, practice another exercise for one of the other parts, and every time come back with another chest exercise, to be followed by any other kind of an exercise, so long as it is not for the part of the body under consideration. The same process must be followed out if it is the neck, arms or any other group of muscles that require specialization. The first, and every other exercise, must be for the specialized part of the body. No doubt you will wonder why this procedure should be followed, so in order to make everything understandable I will explain this to you.

In one of my other chapters I explained how the blood is always drawn to the center of activity. This is the natural method of repletion and absorption. Now after an exercise has been done, the blood continues to circulate over the stimulated area in a greater quantity in order to reconstruct the tissue. One thing I have not explained is this. If you practice any movement until you are fatigued you will deplete your energies so that this process will not be properly performed. Fatigue is brought about by over-relaxation and contraction of the muscle fibers. They continue to contract until the nerve source is not capable of vibrating its electric life through the tissue, and this also lessens the quantity of the blood supply, and thereby deprives the muscles of their nourishing fuel. If you notice the color of the skin you will see that it has become white, just as the face of a person becomes blanched from a mental shock. That is why it is wrong to work or exercise any muscle to the stage where fatigue has set in. As I have previously stated, the natural function of the blood is to replenish, but everything has a limit, and as long as you keep within that limit, which is expressed as being comfortably tired, you can build up continuously. If you go the limit on an exercise that is all you will be able to do, and the reaction of this effort will make itself felt in the rest of the body. By cutting down well within your limit you will both build up and conserve, and while you are practicing an exercise for some other part of the body, nature is doing her work well, carrying away the broken down tissues and leaving its reserve supply for further necessity. This is why it is that by training on the plan I have explained a body builder can keep coming back to his one center of specialization and continue to build up. As you practice in this way observe the change of the skin. It will turn a healthy pink, and you will feel the warm glow of the blood as it suffuses the muscles. In this manner I have exercised for hours at a stretch, always coming back to the one part that I was specializing upon. I never tired, but finished full of pep. Of course, I was somewhat stronger than the average, which enabled me to stand by my practicing so long. Just the same, I was obliged to specialize upon different groups of muscles like any other body builder, who had in view a well-balanced physique.

The man who seems to have the most trouble is the small boned man, and the greyhound type. There appears to be an accepted belief that a man who has small bones cannot build up to any considerable size. The same belief exists with the greyhound type. They find it hard to believe that slabs of muscle can be created upon themselves to fill out their frames. I do not consider these two types as one, as the majority of people do. The greyhound type is invariably the tall, slender, hungry looking individual, who appears to have nothing hanging on his frame. Many men in this group have large bones, but the meat is missing. The small boned man is often a neat looking individual, particularly if he is short. Of the two I find the small boned man much easier to build up than the greyhound type. But, there is no doubt that both of them find the going much harder than their more robust brothers. At that I find that the small boned man is inclined to be a little unreasonable in his demands. He allows figures to overrule certain conditions that he forgets to take into consideration. He will go to a show, and see a fine, big looking fellow, with a 17-inch biceps and a 46-inch chest, who sweeps him completely off his feet with admiration. Right there he wants to be built just like that man. On going home he is almost discouraged to find that his biceps measure only 12 inches and his chest around 36 inches. Still, he will plug away, and maybe get a 15-inch arm and a 40-inch chest, and finally decides there is no use for him to try any more to get that 17-inch biceps. He says it can't be done. In his desire for that 17-inch arm he does not realize that his 15-inch arm is as entirely in proportion to his weight, as is the 17-inch arm of the other man. However, even getting the 17-inch arm can be done. When I commenced heavy training, after putting in years on other athletic work, I had only a 7-inch wrist, and weighed 147 pounds stripped. When I finished I weighed

200 pounds and had a 17½-inch biceps and 47-inch normal chest. Carl Moerke has an 18-inch biceps and a wrist measurement of only a little more than 7 inches. Thomas Inch, the famous English strong man, with a wrist measurement that does not measure 7 inches, developed his body to an enormous degree. His biceps became about 20 inches and chest around 50 inches. Arthur Dandurand, the Canadian Sandow, has a beautifully proportioned arm that measures 17 inches at the biceps, but his wrist is only 7½ inches. In fact, I could name many such examples, where men of small bones developed their body to an extraordinary degree. As a general rule, the small boned man makes the prettiest muscular picture. Now the greyhound type is absolutely a different proposition. His muscles generally present a hungry, stringy appearance, that makes a man feel he has nothing on which to build. He has the appearance of a barren field. The one thing I do find missing about the man with the lean muscles is the entire absence of any interstitial fat. This condition of flesh is very necessary in fertilizing the muscles. In fact, it is an ingredient of exceptional value. The word interstitial means "in between the tissues," and between the fibrous tissues of the muscles this fat secretes itself. The stronger the man, the greater quantity of interstitial fat will he have. This it is which gives his muscles that smooth, silky appearance so often seen, but not so generally understood. Therefore, the greyhound type has to find a method that will create this natural fertilizer. He has two factors to consider, diet and exercise. Ordinarily, I do not pay particular attention to diet. As long as a man is normally healthy and fit, he should allow his stomach to be his guide, but of course, not make a glutton of himself. In this case, the greyhound type should be considered an exception, and by studying the various foods he is able to provide his body with the nutriment that is converted into musculature by exercise, and the other particles not absorbed in this way are carried

by the blood stream to the various parts of the body, to become secreted between the tissues, as interstitial fat.

You no doubt have often heard trainers speak of an athlete training until he goes stale. This is a condition brought about from too vigorous training, in which the muscles are trained raw. Just so raw that the interstitial fat has been absorbed. This causes a reaction upon the nervous system also, which makes the athlete become just "a bunch of nerves."

I have noticed that many of the lean subjects develop into the type of men classified as "raw boney," and while he does not secure the exceptional measurements, yet his muscles seem to be a mass of cords. He becomes one of the cordy muscled type who has as the foundation of his ability very thick ligaments. This type often displays a thickness around the joints, and the owner generally becomes exceptionally strong.

Apart from a special application of diet in the case of the greyhound class, there is a triple method of specialization that can be used by the small bone type, as well as the lean type. However, this is only after they have grounded themselves for a while on a regular all-round system of body culture.

The first thing we know that is desired is size, or, I might better say, space. This is absolutely necessary because as a general rule, the type of men that we are now considering are rarely broad of shoulder, deep of chest, or thick of limb, so we have to develop these conditions. To do this, we must pick out the parts of the body that are most likely to aid us. It does not take long to decide after a physical survey that the back, chest, and thighs are the three parts best suited by nature for our purpose. From now on the men who fall in these two classes must concentrate on broadening their backs, deepening their chests, and rounding their thighs. As this is done a greater space is created on which heavier slabs of muscle can be built. The building up of these three parts will certainly help to make the bodily appearance of any man more massive. I found in many cases that it does not call for any remarkable change on the tape measure around these parts to increase the bodyweight at least ten pounds; but the supposition that these three parts of the body alone when fully developed will build up the rest of the muscles in proportion, is not true. I have seen many athletes with a fine chest who have a poor neck, and men with broad shoulders have a weak lower back. Others, with good thighs, have poor arms and calf muscles. By training on these triple parts, good abdominal and lower back development is apt to be created, along with better formed hips. The neck, forearms, biceps, deltoids and calves will not be developed in proportion, and specialization, as I explained earlier in this chapter, will be found necessary.

I cannot understand why anyone should become worried because they have only a small wrist. The man who has a big hand is likely to have a large wrist. If a man had a large hand and only a small wrist it would be very different, as the difference would be disproportionate. Just the same, the man with the big wrist has to build up his arm in proportion to the boney structure he possesses. Anyhow, why worry over what the other fellow has? You have a fixed object in your mind that you want to build up certain proportions, so concentrate upon the subject. Don't get the idea in your head that because you have a weight in your hands it alone will give you the results if you simply go through a number of repetitions in a certain position. It has been explained long ago that the mind moves the mass. The thousands of nerve centers in the body that are directed by the brain control the activity of the whole muscular system, and mentally, your movements can be registered as fixed determination or arrant listlessness. The first gives power, the second lacks power. Wherever you concentrate your mind, your nerve energies will center, and a greater resistance is evidenced. Mental concentration draws all the natural resources forward in mutual sympathy to intensify the functioning duties of the motive muscles. Therefore, it is readily seen what is meant when a pupil is advised to concentrate strongly upon the physical movements that form the exercise.

Of course, there is no use in any of us kidding ourselves that we can all be big men with enormous proportions. That would not be logical or even desirable. Take it this way. If you stand only 5' 3" and if it was possible for you to weigh 225 pounds, all solid muscle, what would you look like? Nothing nice. You would only make a monstrosity of yourself. You can be equally as strong by being proportionate. I do not see what necessity there is for everyone to want to be a Gorner or a Steinbach. All well and good, if your physical possibilities throw you in their class; but talking with the fact in mind, that all cannot be two hundred pounders, we must realize the impossibility of this. Of course, I know it would be great if we could be as good as these men by building up from a natural angle, but we cannot. Build yourself up to the best of your ability and be satisfied to be a good man in your class. Charles Schaffer was the Gorner of the 112 pound class, just the same as Marineau was the Gorner of the lightweights. If you are only 5' 3" tall, and weigh 150 pounds stripped, with a 15½" neck, 15" biceps, 14½" calf, and a 39" normal chest, you will be a pretty husky chap. Of course, there are men much heavier than that, but I am talking about a condition that is well within your reach, and which will make of the man an unusually capable physical machine. When a man reaches the height of 5' 6", he can scale from 175 pounds up to 200, and safely combine the dual attributes of size with strength. Such a man is a dynamo of power, and his measurements can all be large and perfectly balanced. A 200-pound man of this type would have to register a 17½" biceps, 18" neck, 47" normal chest, a 16½" calf, and a 25½" thigh. These measurements will give you an idea of what a man can work up to according to his class, and still remain out of the phenomena order. Look how well balanced Gorner is. His great strength is the result of highly balanced attributes. There have been many men much larger than Gorner, but not half as strong, which is a positive proof that they lacked balance somewhere. I dislike phenomenally built men; it really does not mean anything. These monstrosities, with twenty-two-inch biceps and calves, with sixty-inch chests, with 22" biceps and calves, with 60" chests, while standing less than 6' in height, do not come within the sphere of the body culturist, who worships a beautifully built body and vigorous strength. I have met them, but none were nearly as strong as I am, and they were unlovely to look upon. If I had to pick out the two biggest men who combined the two qualities, shape and strength, in a proper balance, I would name George Hackenschmidt and Herman Gorner as the finest combination ever produced. Size, strength, speed and physical loveliness they possessed, without registering any unusual bodyweight.

Hackenschmidt had only ordinary measurements with which to start, but right living and intelligent exercise on the bar bell progressive principle made him what he was, and is today. No matter if your wrist is only 6", and your weight 125 pounds, you can build yourself into as fine a specimen of manhood as any other of your own height. Height should rule more than bone size, and always bear in mind what one man has secured for himself you can get also. This may not be absolutely true, but it is true that you can come near enough to him to invite a favorable comparison.

CHAPTER XX
WHAT IS MAN'S LIMIT IN WEIGHT-LIFTING?

How quickly that question will make followers of the sport of weight lifting prick up their ears and listen. It is an eternal question and one that is asked in every line of sport. No doubt long before Samson carried away the Gates of Gath, and positively ever since, many have asked this question, "What is the ultimate limit of man's strength?" Everything has its limits, no matter whether it is a machine or a human being running a race, a limit is always reached; but what we are greatly interested in, is how far we can go before the limit is reached. When Sandow made his first record in the bent press of two hundred and sixty-five pounds, the world thought the pinnacle was reached. Then along came Saxon and he shattered it by well over a hundred pounds. He did not receive any extra aid from any special lifting apparatus in any of his lifts. He could do as well with the weights of any other lifter. It is sometimes claimed that special apparatus is always used when record performances are made. The actual truth is that the weight lifter will always have to rely upon his speed and strength. His success lies within himself, as explained in the chapter "Where is the Science in Lifting Weights?" I do not deny that there are many types of bars which help him a little, but these are often the undoing of the athletes. The heavier the weight, the greater the rebound in a very springy bar. A cambered bar is useful in bent pressing a weight. It helps to kill the roll of the bar and the tipping in the hand, but neither Sandow nor Saxon used a cambered bar, nor did Gorner, Giroux, Cadine, or Rigoulot in their dead lifts with one and two hands. Not one' of these men used any special bars for their snatch, swing, or clean and jerk lifts, just the regular plate loading bells, and in some of the lifts they used the old type shot loading bell. All of which goes to prove that the weight lifter has not, up to date, received any really valuable aid from the change made in bars. Any records I have made were made with the ordinary plate loading bell, the shot loading bell or a combination of both, and mostly with thick handle bars, excepting the swing when I employed a "back hang." Still there is no doubt in my mind that the cambered bar is very helpful in one and two hand dead lifting, and in the bent press. Some lifters can use this same bar to a greater advantage in the one hand snatch, and one hand clean and jerk. What I mean is, that the mechanical strides made in weight lifting apparatus are not as great as those made in some other sports. For example, the new ball used in baseball has greater liveliness and is calculated to increase its flight thirty or forty feet over the ball used a few years back, and this has naturally increased the number of home runs. At one time, hammer throwers swung a blacksmith's sledge hammer. Now a ball hammer has a specially constructed handle and revolves on ball bearings. The weight lifting game is entirely different. The lifter cannot get up a great momentum with a weight and let it go the way a hammer thrower does. He always has to overcome the resistance of the weight, and sustain it in order to make a lift.

Laboratory research has done a lot for other sports, but nothing for weight lifting so far. Nevertheless, I can make a bar that could revolutionize weight lifting; at any rate increase the abilities of the lifter by twenty to twenty-five per cent on all lifts but the military press lift, and it would be more legitimate than the "western roll" used in high jumping and which has caused so much controversy.

However, that has nothing to do with my subject, analyzing the possibilities of the strong man as they exist today. Quite a number of years ago I drew up a tabulated list of records on various lifts, naming certain poundages that I believed would be reached within the period of a few years by lifters in the three classes that I scheduled. Most of my weight lifting friends and followers raised their brows in amazement, for as they expressed themselves, they were not used to hearing me talk outside the realms of possibility. Some were kind enough to say that if they had not known me so well they would have doubted my sobriety when I made the schedule. I will agree that they did appear staggering, as they were way out of sight at that time in comparison with the then existing records. I had many reasons for my prophecy, which I have explained in other chapters. However, the World War broke out and everything was set back, but in the few years of post-war reconstruction most of the records I had named have been equaled and in many cases surpassed. What is more remarkable, many of these records have been knocked off their pedestals by lighter men than I took into consideration at that time. In those days a middleweight was from one hundred and fifty-four pounds to one hundred and sixty-one pounds, and a lightweight scaled from one hundred and forty-seven pounds up to one hundred and fifty-four. Now a lightweight can only scale from one hundred and twenty-six pounds to one hundred and forty pounds, and the middleweight follows up to one hundred and fifty-four pounds. I kept the chart of figures and thinking you will find them interesting, I will lay them before you. But I want you to bear in mind when surveying the records, that they were listed according to the bodyweights of that time. Another thing I want to bring before your attention in respect to bodyweight, is the difference in the European class weights and ours. All of the European bodyweights are a few pounds heavier than ours in the same class, which according to our figures would throw many of their best men up into the next bodyweight class. So please always remember that when making your comparison. It is really this vexed bodyweight question that has developed the belief that the Europeans are much better than the

American strength athletes. When you have concluded reading this chapter, you will be both surprised and proud to see how the American post-war weight lifter has forged to the front, and the favorable comparison he makes with our foreign strong men.

It seems like a hard job for me to get started to give you the promised list, but I feel I have so much to talk about that I believe may interest you, that I find it hard to include everything in the space of these chapters. Anyway, here goes. Look these figures over, just so that you will not feel the shock of the high marks so badly. I have placed an asterisk alongside of each record that has been either equaled or surpassed.

Heavyweight class. Two Hands Continental Jerk *425 pounds. Two Hands Clean and Jerk *375 pounds. Two Hands Snatch *270 pounds. Two Hands Anyhow 475 pounds. One Hand Clean and Jerk 265 pounds. One Hand Snatch *235 pounds. One Hand Swing *220 pounds. One Hand Anyhow *400 pounds.

Old Middleweight class (161 pounds). Two Hands Continental Jerk *340 pounds. Two Hands Clean and Jerk 300 pounds. Two Hands Snatch *230 pounds. Two Hands Anyhow 375 pounds. One Hand Clean and Jerk 240 pounds. One Hand Snatch *200 pounds. One Hand Swing *180 pounds. One Hand Anyhow 325 pounds.

Old Lightweight class (147 pounds). Two Hand Continental Jerk *275 pounds. Two Hands Clean and Jerk *250 pounds. Two Hands Snatch *200 pounds. Two Hands Any- how *320' pounds. One Hand Clean and Jerk *200 pounds. One Hand Snatch 175 pounds. One Hand Swing 165 pounds. One Hand Anyhow *265 pounds.

You will see that of the twenty-four records listed, sixteen have been equaled or surpassed. The remaining eight are not so far out of sight as you may imagine. The fact is that by the time you have this book in your hands some of the eight records will have fallen. Already, they are dangerously threatened. The records that are likely to remain untouched longest are the Two Hands Anyhow, and the One Hand Anyhow, in the middleweight class. The sole reason for this is, that the bent press is the principal part of these lifts, especially in the One Hand Anyhow. In the Two Hands Anyhow, quite a few perform the lift by jerking the weight overhead with two hands and then transferring it to one hand; then by reaching down and picking up a dumbbell, or kettle bell, and pressing overhead the lift is concluded. As I was saying, the principal part of these two lifts is the bent press, and just now we haven't many good middleweight bent press men. If any man at the present time can do either of these lifts, Fournier is the man, He is a master of the bent press and the two hands jerk and can handle a rare poundage in either lift, which makes him quite capable of equaling these marks, if he trained for them. He is much below the old middleweight limit, scaling one hundred and fifty-four pounds, but at that weight he has bent pressed from the shoulder and held at arms' length a living weight of over three hundred pounds. As I said in another chapter, to bent press a man is easier than a weight, but the fact remains he held the weight at arms' length after raising it, which proves that he has the sustaining power, which means a great deal in the Two Hands Anyhow. I have seen him jerk with two hands three hundred pounds three times in succession. We have seen that he can hold over three hundred pounds at arms' length in one hand, and jerk three hundred pounds easily with two hands, therefore there should be no trouble for him to transfer two hundred and eighty pounds to one hand, and raise a hundred pounds with the other hand, with a little training. Then there was Kosakwitz, who at only one hundred and forty-five pounds, found no difficulty in jerking with two hands over three hundred pounds, and he too was a great bent press man. Even Maxick was a great bent press man. Although it is not so well known, at one time he trained to lift double his bodyweight in that style, and in training succeeded, which means he was able to raise at least two hundred and ninety-four pounds in the bent press. Business in the first place, and the outbreak of the war in the second place prevented him from obtaining an official record. His wonderful two arm jerk of three hundred and twenty-two pounds, at a bodyweight of less than one hundred and fifty pounds shows the wonderful ability he possessed. Had he been trained for those two lifts he would have been able to surpass those marks. Tromp Van Diggelen, who brought out Maxick, believed that his protégé could have raised four hundred pounds in the Two Hands Anyhow. Time was when people thought the records made by the famous veterans of the past would never be equaled; but history, in repeating itself, has completely eclipsed nearly all of these marks. The great prodigies of man power do not come often, but they do come, which proves the saying that "where there is one good man, there will be another."

In the Two Hands Continental Jerk, we find the mark of four hundred and twenty-five pounds not only equaled but beaten by the great Austrian butcher, Swoboda, and the South African German, Gorner, even went higher than the crack Vienna iron man. The mark in the Two Hands Clean and Jerk is equaled by no less than four men, Gorner, Alzin, Rigoulot and Stein- born. Rigoulot is given credit in training with a mark of three hundred and seventy-seven pounds, and the terrific weight of four hundred pounds is predicted in French lifting circles for this great Parisian weight heaver. I have also heard it said that if Gorner could develop the same skill as Rigoulot, four hundred and fifty pounds would not be beyond his limit in this lift. It is a fact that Gorner is not as skillful a lifter as Rigoulot, Cadine or Stein- born. Like Swoboda and Alzin, he relies solely upon his prodigious strength. The mention of Alzin brings to my mind no reason why he could not make the grade in the first named lift. He is undoubtedly the heaviest man in the game. His bodyweight given to me just recently is in the neighborhood of three hundred and twenty-six pounds. I know some time ago, when I first heard of him, he gave his weight at two hundred and eighty-nine pounds stripped. He is tall and seems to have unlimited man power, and it would be interesting to know what he could do in a trial on the Two Hands Continental Jerk.

The affection that our present day iron manipulators have for the fast lifts quickly wrecked the scheduled mark on the Two Hands Snatch, and it looks as though it is in for a real beating. Steinborn was the first man to draw American attention to the one and two hands snatch and prove their great possibilities as I had outlined them, when he made a mark of two hundred and sixty pounds with the two hands. Previously, Josef Stienbach had done two hundred and sixty-four and three quarter pounds, and most lifting authorities had thought the highest mark was then reached in that lift. Indeed, one famous European when speaking to me said, that it had taken twenty centuries to produce a man like Stienbach, and we would never see his lifts equaled, because he had the great combination of speed, size and strength. His press lifts I admitted appeared to be out of sight, but I told him that he would be surprised someday. No doubt he was when he heard a man like Steinborn, who is a considerably smaller man than the Vienna Cafe proprietor, had put up two hundred and sixty pounds, and Rondi the German, was given the world's record with two hundred and seventy pounds two years before Steinborn made his record in Philadelphia. It is also a fact that Steinborn snatched the same bar as Rondi, in an impromptu contest in Germany. We find that Hackenschmidt had scored a mark of two hundred and fifty-five pounds, eclipsing the big Vienna butcher, Swoboda, whose best stood at two hundred and forty-three pounds. The great Louis Vasseur, had an official mark of two hundred and sixty pounds. Giroux and Alzin, both stopped at two hundred and fifty-six pounds. Ernest Cadine, when weighing well under two hundred pounds, made a fine mark of two hundred and fifty-nine and a half pounds. Then Rigoulot came forward and eclipsed the former Olympic champion, with a mark of two hundred and seventy-one pounds and finally he hung up two hundred and seventy-seven pounds. This figure beat Gorner's record of two hundred and seventy-five and a half pounds. Just recently Rigoulot made another attempt to break his record on that lift, but just failed at two hundred and eighty-six pounds. There is no doubt that this is marvelous lifting, and they claim that the Parisian wonder has set his heart on reaching three hundred pounds in the Two Hands Snatch, before he says he is through. On the fourth lift, the Two Hands Anyhow, while no one has broken Saxon's record of four hundred and forty-eight pounds, yet I believe it is only a matter of making the attempt. I feel quite sure that any of the following four men, Gorner, Moerke, Steinborn, and Alzin, could beat the mark if they tried. Gorner made four hundred and forty and three-quarter pounds in this lift in an impromptu attempt. Judging by his other lifts, I would not put five hundred pounds past this giant. Arthur Saxon stated years ago, that if Gorner would train on the bent press, he would beat all of Saxon's own records, as he admitted that Gorner—who was a younger member of the same club—was a much stronger man than he. I quite believe Henry Steinborn could equal that mark, without even employing the bent press. It is a fact that four hundred pounds in the Two Hands Anyhow, is way below his best. The One Hand Clean and Jerk has been closely approached by both Gorner and Gaessler in practice. Gorner has jerked from the shoulder with the right arm, two hundred and sixty-four and a half pounds, and Gaessler has a clean all the way record of two hundred and fifty-one pounds, although it is claimed that Arthur Saxon lifted two hundred and sixty- seven pounds, which beats my figure. When I consider the ability of the snatch and swing lifter of to-day, it is a wonder to me that the mark of two hundred and sixty-five pounds has not been broken before now. Although the one hand snatch record has not made much progress since Vasseur did his stuff, yet I have heard that Steinborn equaled my figure while training in New York. I believe it is quite possible for him. One time he was quite serious in wanting to make a bet that he would give five dollars for every pound he snatched below two hundred and thirty pounds, providing anyone present would give him ten dollars for every pound he snatched over two hundred and thirty pounds. They all seemed quite satisfied that they would be handling the losing end, so the contest never took place. We find that Rigoulot in his match against Cadine, scored two hundred and twenty-three pounds. If he could score a splendid total like that in a match of ten lifts, where a man must of necessity conserve his strength; what would he do on a single attempt ? I would say two hundred and forty pounds. On the One Hand Swing, Gorner gets credit for breaking my schedule of two hundred and twenty pounds, by swinging two hundred and twenty and a half pounds. Just by half a pound. Yes, but I would like to impress upon you the fact, that when he created that record, he swung with a lead dumb-bell. Of all the unwieldy objects to handle, a lead weight is the worst. You may think that there is no difference. Well, just try it. Anyhow, a spherical dumbbell is a very bad implement to swing, as the weight is distributed over too large an area. It is hard to say what he would do employing a back hang style, where the weight is more compact, and one end being heavier than the other enables the dumb-bell to be more easily controlled. Rigoulot is creeping up to the mark too, so we must not be surprised at what follows. On the last named lift, the One Hand Anyhow, I think we can rightfully give Arthur Saxon the honor of equaling the schedule. He actually lifted four hundred pounds in London before witnesses, but just as he was straightening up beneath the weight, some of the miscellaneous weights that had been tied to the bar, fell off. Still, that does not alter the fact that the weight had already been pressed. What he actually sustained, was a total of three hundred and eighty-six and three-quarter pounds, as verified by the scales.

This analysis of the heavyweight class, substantially proves their ability to equal the marks that I prophesized for them, and as we continue with the other two classes, further facts will be advanced that will prove to you what really has happened in the world of weights since I made that schedule, and that will give you a more definite idea of what we can expect in the future.

In the middleweight class, you will notice that the schedule was given at the old bodyweight, therefore let us still continue to consider the marks of men within that limit, and see just what has been done. You will be surprised to see what the athlete has accomplished in the lighter bodyweight classes. I think it is only fair that we should consider them this way in order to make a fairer comparison with our own athletes, for as I have previously remarked, the European bodyweight classes are heavier than ours. Just for example, Aeschman, the Swiss crack middleweight, scales around one hundred and sixty pounds, and when he made his attempt at two hundred and ninety-seven and a half pounds in the Two Hands Clean and Jerk, he weighed one hundred and sixty-five pounds. Commencing with the first lift, which I have marked at three hundred and forty pounds, Maxick at about one hundred and fifty pounds jerked in the Two Hands Continental style three hundred and twenty-two pounds. I came next at one hundred and fifty-four pounds with three hundred and ten pounds. Both Maxick and myself have beaten our official marks in training. I was informed that Maxick did three hundred and forty pounds, and while I did not have my arms perfectly straight underneath the weight,

I managed to sustain three hundred and thirty-eight pounds. Of course this is not a complete lift, but if my time had not been so much occupied with wrestling, I believe I would have broken the mark myself before I had left the middleweight ranks. However, keeping within the present middleweight limit I believe Fournier could train up to that mark, as I have seen him jerk well over three hundred pounds in ordinary training, without concentrating on that particular lift. In fact, the only time I ever saw him perform the Two Hands Continental Jerk, was when I suggested it to him. Within the European limit, I knew two men who made the grade. Unfortunately these boys were casualties of the late war.

The Two Hands Clean and Jerk is being badly crowded although not yet equaled. It is due for a tumble any time. At one hundred and fifty-four pounds I cleaned two hundred and seventy- two pounds, and my pupil Fournier is crowding the same mark at the same bodyweight, hanging up two hundred and seventy pounds to his credit. At a little heavier bodyweight which put me in our heavy middleweight class, but as a middleweight, according to the Olympic bodyweight scale, I succeeded with two hundred and eighty-two pounds. Kikkas, of Estonia, recently made a fine performance coming close to the scheduled mark with two hundred and eighty and a half pounds. However, his mark did not stand long. Vibert, of France, jumped into the setting with a scant lead of a half pound. Not long afterwards the fine Swiss middleweight, Aeschman, crowded into the limelight with two hundred and eighty-seven pounds to his credit. Now Holland, a country little heard of in weight lifting, has produced an amateur in Verhyen, who is only three pounds behind my hypothetical mark; namely, two hundred and ninety-seven pounds. As I said earlier in the chapter, Aeschman just failed with two hundred and ninety-seven and a half pounds, so you see this mark is not going to stay unequalled long.

One record that brought forth quite a debate was the mark I gave for the Two Hands Snatch in the middleweight class. They all calmly told me I was crazy. Two hundred pounds was the limit. Now here is the way I figured it out. At one hundred and fifty-four pounds I could two hands snatch two hundred pounds and that lift was one I seldom practiced. I could Military Press any time with two arms two hundred and thirty pounds, and I figured a man in the lighter classes than the heavyweights should be able to snatch with two hands whatever he could Military Press with both hands. So far most snatchers are poor press lifters, but good press lifters can usually snatch what they press. Of course, you may say why did I not do so. The only excuse I can offer was that I never cared for the lift. Then again, I do not want to talk about myself, as I would far rather talk about what others have done to prove my prophecies, although I have made mention of myself on two or three occasions. Again, I will have to remark about myself as I did perform that poundage in practice. I believed others could do better than myself, as I never really concentrated on weight lifting training like many of the other men I am recording. Actually my feats were more the result of my strength gained from exercise than the result of constant practice aimed at enabling me to break records. To get back to my subject let me say that the two hundred pound mark was easily beaten. Fournier went past it. Then Neuland, who rates as a lightweight in Europe, sent the record soaring up to two hundred and twenty pounds. Aeschman beat it with a mark of two hundred and twenty-two pounds, which is near enough to prove that what I did in practice will be done by many others.

Previously I explained why neither the One Hand Anyhow or the Two Hands Anyhow marks have not been equaled, so I will pass these lifts over and talk about the One Hand Clean. At the present time no one has come near the mark set by Maxick of two hundred and thirty-eight pounds, which is only two pounds below the schedule on this lift. Bicheel, of Switzerland, holds the present amateur record in both the light and middleweight class, with a mark of two hundred and nine pounds, although I have heard that he has since succeeded with two hundred and sixteen pounds. Maurice De Riaz, as a middleweight, was given credit for doing two hundred and twenty-three pounds. In the One Hand Snatch a former partner of Maxick told me he saw the Bavarian wonder do two hundred pounds, which equals my scheduled mark. Others are coming close as is proven by the record made by Neuland, of Estonia, with one hundred and eighty-one and a half pounds, which was later pulled down by the Austrian, Trelfny, with one hundred and eighty-three pounds only to be superseded by Zinner, of Germany, with a mark of one hundred and eighty-seven pounds.

The one hand swing brings the British lifter into prominence, and I am given to understand that the fine English swing lifter, C. V. Wheeler, equaled in a practice swing my named mark of one hundred and eighty pounds. Aston, another British swing lifter at a bodyweight that would qualify him for the class where the mark was set up, came only two pounds short of the mark, using the old style swing.

The lightweight division has come to the front strongly in vindicating my schedule. Kosakwitz, at one hundred and forty- five pounds, performed three hundred and eight pounds in the Two Hands Continental Jerk. Of course, he is five pounds heavier than our present lightweight scale allows, yet he is about right for the European limit and is two pounds under the old lightweight limit. This great little Russian went thirty-three pounds over my selection and Marineau has equaled two hundred and seventy-five pounds at a bodyweight of less than one hundred and forty pounds. We find the mark of two hundred and fifty pounds for the two hands Clean and Jerk almost as badly shattered as the first named lift. Marineau has done two hundred and sixty- six pounds in my presence. Reenfrank, of France, did two hundred and fifty-two pounds, then his countryman, Arnout, did two hundred and fifty-three pounds. The final coup was supplied by De Haas, the Belgium, with two hundred and sixty-nine and a half pounds. Nineteen and a half pounds in excess of my mark. Siegmund Klein, who would have come within the old lightweight limit, goes over two hundred and fifty pounds, and I expect to see him do quite a lot more. The Two Hands Snatch mark has taken a good beating. Neuland, of Estonia, and Arnout, of France, are tie at two hundred and twenty pounds. We must not forget that when Maxick was within the lightweight limit he could wreck some of the scheduled marks. In the Two Hands Anyhow, for instance, three hundred and twenty pounds would not stop him. A year ago, Marineau claimed to have performed three hundred and eighteen pounds by employing the Bent Press as part of the lift. Being such a master lifter I know quite well that he could equal three hundred and twenty pounds. The one lift I thought I had made a little high was the One Hand Clean and Jerk. I fully believed that the mark would be reached, but I figured it would be some time before this was accomplished. However, the great little Swiss, Bicheel, backed up my belief with a real lift of two hundred and nine pounds some time ago, and just to prove that wonders will never cease, Hans Haas came forward with an astounding lift of two hundred and twenty pounds.

The One Hand Snatch record lacks ten pounds of my record, but it will be reached. Neuland has performed with one hundred and sixty-five pounds and promises to lift much more. The One Hand Swing is not so good. Cobly, an English lifter, has done one hundred and forty-five pounds, but I believe that Monte Saldo within the old limit did somewhere around one hundred and fifty- four pounds. Incidentally he was the first man in the world to ever swing more than his own weight. These last two lifts show the slowest progress, but the fast lifters are invading the ranks of the lighter class and like the One Hand Clean and Jerk, the selected marks will be equaled. The One Hand Anyhow of two hundred and sixty-five pounds has been equaled by Marineau not long ago, and Fournier also made the same poundage before he stepped into the heavier ranks of the middleweights.

Not a great many years ago, all the records that compose this schedule were considered impossible, but as you see, most of them have already been shelved, and the rest are scheduled to go at any time now. This goes to show that the limitations of man are governed by the times. Within the last few years we have marched fast, and the records have kept pace. Undoubtedly they will go higher yet in every class as new apparatus is introduced and perfected in the game as it has been in other sports. The sport of weight lifting is just in its infancy, and much can be predicted for its future. What the actual limits will be, time alone can tell. I once set a standard that was deemed impossible, but within a short time my marks have been proven beatable, and I will say that whatever the marks of today may be, the records of tomorrow will eclipse them all.

CHAPTER XXI
WHY HOME EXERCISE IS BEST

You may have heard would-be body culturists say, "Aw gee, how can I train ? There is no gymnasium around here, and any way if there was, I couldn't afford it." Actually, hundreds of young men have presented this problem to me, hoping that I would be able to solve the little difficulty for them. It is quite natural for any person to consider exercise and a gymnasium at the same time. As I have said at different times, it depends on what you are after. If it is games or calisthenics, all right. By all means become a member of a gymnastic class. They will certainly teach you to become good at the game you prefer, and this will help to keep you healthy and fit at the same time. Calisthenics will freshen you up and keep you normally fit, but if it is your whole body you want to build up to a stage of perfection, then it is an entirely different proposition. Of course, there are exercise rooms in all gymnasiums to which you can go and seclude yourself, but they do not always have the proper apparatus at hand for the body culturist to use. Of course, there is always the congeniality of companionship, but I have found that this is often very embarrassing, especially to the man who is under developed or too fat. There is always somebody willing to pass remarks, which even when made in fun, go a long way to diminish enthusiasm. Often a man is too conscious of his condition, and what he requires is encouragement, not to be made the object of fun no matter how good natured it may be. This may give you the idea that I do not approve of gymnasiums. On the contrary, I do approve of them, but if you want to do any body building, do it at home. Of course, if you know an instructor who has an unusual interest in his clients and understands progressive body building, then that is different. He will be a great help if you can afford to pay for his services. Unfortunately many cannot. Others live in the country, or do not have the time at their disposal. There is nothing in the world that can overcome these little difficulties like home training. As long as you have space in your bedroom to spread your arms level with your shoulders, and stretch out to arms' length overhead, you have all the room necessary to train. Three or four nights a week training just before you retire will fix you up, and if you have more time to spare, you can devote some of it at the gym to your favorite game, be it boxing, wrestling, or handball; but if you are deeply interested in building up your body to its finest state of perfection you will be apt to give more time to your training than just three or four periods a week. Home is more convenient, and there you have no one to bother you. If you can get another friend to train with you that will be fine, but more than one only detracts the others from their training, as conversation is bound to waste the precious minutes.

First, what a body builder or health seeker wants, is an outfit that will give him the best results. I can honestly say that there is nothing that can equal a bar bell outfit. All that is required is a set of graded plates of iron that will enable the home exerciser to increase his poundage as he improves in size and strength, with a handle bar about five feet long, dumb-bell handles, and kettle- weight handles—then he is all set to go. These sets can be bought to suit the purse of the individual. If a person wants to build up in size and strength enough to make his appearance a little better than the average, and yet feel vigorously fit, an outfit weighing from one hundred to two hundred pounds is enough. If it is great strength and muscular proportions that he desires, then he will require a heavier set. The next step is to be sure to obtain the best instructions from a teacher in whom you feel that you have faith. When you have these all together and settled, you will be surprised to find how this will convert your room into a gymnasium of your own.

As I look back over the years, my mind dwells fondly upon the little bedroom that has long been treasured in my memory. Within those four walls I spent many hours struggling for a better body. It was right there that I fought my battles and won my victories. No matter how hopeless some things may have appeared during those days, I always saw the turn at the end of the road. How I loved those days. My parents took great pride in my healthy body and unusual strength, but they began to think I was too enthusiastic when I began to tow in weights. Oh, no, my dear friend, we were not so lucky then as to have the convenient plate loading bells that you have today. They were all solid weights, or lumps of iron, and they were terribly expensive. Anyhow, my mother thought to scare me out of the idea, and told me I would have to go up in the attic and live. Well, I went up to the attic all right and carried all my stuff with me. Mother would shake her head and dad would grin. I first got a pair of dumb-bells, then a heavy iron part of an old axle, a block weight, and a ninety pound dumb-bell. I used the latter for a bar bell as well as a dumb-bell by catching hold of the outside on the big nuts and pushing it overhead with both hands. I pinned my exercises on the wall and started out. Bit by bit I accumulated my outfits, and a proud boy was I when I surveyed my first plate loading bar bell. Pictures began to appear upon the bare walls in neat formation, and on the winter nights I gazed upon my ideals and inspirations and plugged away. Bare floors meant nothing to me and, oh yes, I had a big cracked mirror, too. I slept on a little camp cot, where I dreamed of my ambitions all night. I kept the place clean myself, and in later years mother would show her friends my little sanctum with pride. I accumulated a little physical culture library, and gradually decorated my room with my outfits, photos, diplomas, medals and other trophies. For years, after I left home, they kept the room just as I had kept it. No one else was allowed to occupy it.

Perhaps the saddest part of it was that my wanderings took me so far away that I never returned to my boyhood home and its treasured memories. For in the meantime death had intervened and broke up my parental home. Still, you see others viewed it as a sacred spot besides myself. I attended gym classes and played all outdoor sports, but it was the environment I was able to build within the four walls of my bedroom that enabled me to concentrate on my exercise training in such a manner as would be impossible elsewhere. It laid the foundation of my athletic success.

You can create your own ideals in home training, without fear of disturbance, just as thousands of others have. You get a hundred times better results. There is no lost motion there, you can concentrate and win.

A little while ago I received a long letter from one of my old chums who had often taken a work-out with me up in my little bedroom. We had not met for about twenty years. He was a little older than I and went out to Australia. He still is an exercise bug. How I would like you to read his letter. He longed for the old days, as we all do, but he remembers best the many happy hours we spent together building ourselves into efficient manhood in that little attic. Proudly he reminded me that the very best specimen of manhood were all home exercise fans, men who did not require elaborate gymnasiums. It is true. Sandow, Maxick, Pullum, MacMahon, Berry, Coulter, Manger, Matysek, Willoughby, Snyder, Klein and a host of others got the foundation and the subsequent results of their marvelous physiques within their bedroom chamber. You can't beat it. Thirty minutes' intensive exercise, a good rub down, and then jump into bed and you will sleep like a rock, waking up with the life coursing through your veins that will make you fit for any emergency.

If you want a forty-four inch chest, a sixteen and a half inch biceps, twenty-five inch thigh, or a sixteen inch calf, don't overlook the value of your own home. It is more economical and result producing, and then you are at home. When winter comes don't be afraid of a little cold atmosphere, it will do you good and help you to pep up.

I know that many of the most famous strong men did all their weight lifting training in their bedrooms. It was within the confines of those four walls that they put up their best poundages.

Nowadays, home training has become recognized by the majority of people as the way to get the very best results in body building. Nowhere else can individual instructions be given to as good an advantage, for every prospective body builder must recognize the fact that no material results can be obtained unless the exercises are laid out to suit the physical requirements of the individual. What suits one person does not suit another, which is one reason why mass drill is only a body toner and not a body builder. Intensive training only, will produce muscular growth and proportionate strength. This method of training requires the knowledge of one who is fully acquainted with the body, and its peculiarities in muscular growth in order to secure the best results for the pupil. In this book I have tried to explain everything about the muscles and their operations, as well as the why's and wherefore's of exercise, how it should be done and what points to most carefully consider. In this way it is possible for everyone to map out a course for himself to suit himself, which is bound to give him the very best results in his home training.

CHAPTER XXII
Do You Know the Sources of Your Vitality?

The title of this chapter asks a question that will make you think a little to answer it in anything like a correct way. No one can really answer the question fully, simply because each day science is unveiling some great bodily essential not previously known; or scientists find out the important relations between certain organisms, all of which should be of great interest to you. Over two thousand years ago, Solomon, among his wise sayings, remarked in reverent awe that the body is wonderfully and fearfully made. In his great wisdom the sage of Israel realized the nature of God's work, but not in the concrete way that the investigations of present day science have made possible for us. Science is a never ending cycle in which each new subject seems to be more interesting than the last. Research sets me athirst all the time to know more of this ingenious body of ours. Bodily comparison and relativity is a wonderful study. While this subject allows us to find out much about the body, to me its greatest value lies in what it enables us to infer. By inference it brings enlightenment on many hithertofore hazy beliefs. Just for example, take "Growth and Development" by Spencer. In it he does not make a single mention of body culture, but growth, as presented in plant and animal life by Spencer, has been of great use to me in my comparisons. The law of relativity, as he expounds it, taught me the first principles of gravity, which I later worked out on a mathematical scale and applied successfully to lifting inanimate objects. Drummond in his "The Ascent of Man" gives much instruction by inference. His lament for the physical neglect of the human race is poignant. In that volume he says, "Time was when every man was an athlete, now to our shame, we have to pay to see one." Since he wrote, the blessings of body culture have been more fully recognized, and today we can see one hundred well built men to every ten of twenty-five years ago. Huxley, Wallace, Darwin and Osbourne all have taught great lessons by explaining the natural changes brought about in the evolution of man. Whether man descended from the apes or not, it is very interesting to note the physical changes that have taken place through the ages in his physical construction. It is only natural that as his method of living changed, it had a lot to do with changing his actual strength. Scientists have not proven that the prehistoric man of the stone age was so physically larger than the modern man. Taking them as a whole, the average stone age man was undoubtedly physically a better specimen. In those days, man lived entirely out of doors and was a hunter from necessity. Things have changed, and a certain proportion of men nowadays spend their time within an office or a store. Naturally, there are certain things that we have lost, but there is a natural law of compensation and where men of prehistoric times were possessed of brute strength, the modern man is possessed of intelligent strength. As mechanical science released us from too much manual effort, mental intelligence acquired for us a system that enabled us to keep our body as perfectly fit as our ancestors. Of course, I cannot go into detail here to prove all this. And I think you would not be as interested in the exact reasons, as you are in the results. But after reading considerable material on the subject of evolution I have come to the conclusion that in physical construction man has changed very little. The greatest changes have been mental. Also various internal organs have been obliged to adopt themselves to the changes made by our changed system of eating. However, this is just another example of the law of compensation. Each loss necessitates a change to compensate for it, just as the principles of exercise enable us to develop all our muscles to the very best of their natural state. I believe that the average body culturist is a better specimen of manhood than the average man of any previous age. The man of by-gone ages hunted, fished, made war, ate and slept, but all that did not make them more powerful, as much as it made them a hardier race by reason of their bodily exposure to the elements. No doubt the slaves who bent their backs under the whips in building the pyramids of Egypt were more powerfully constructed than the prehistoric man by reason of their excessive labors. It took a good man to survive the brutalities of that period. History gives plenty of evidence of this. The first half of the seventh century B. C. saw the Median revolt against Assyrian world domination, and it was during this calamity that the slaves held in captivity availed themselves of the opportunity to escape, which they did successfully. They developed into a formidable war-like race, finally enlisting under Alexander the Great, and played the most important part in all the brilliant campaigns of that great leader.

This is a little off the subject, but I merely mention it as a point of evidence.

Man in his transitory stages of evolution has lost the need for some things. For instance, the troublesome appendix which the modern person finds he can get on as well without. In fact, many physicians believe that he is better off without it. A survey of the United States Army statistics, estimating the physical standard of recruits during the World War, show an amazing percentage of soldiers who were minus the appendix. With the prehistoric man this tract was necessary as an organ of digestion. Its use is not entirely eliminated by the modern man; during infancy it functions, but not afterwards, and this is the reason why it is dangerous, as it allows matter to become secreted within itself and may become infected. It is claimed that this tract is less dangerous in an individual who follows a vigorous occupation, as for instance, laborers, blacksmiths, or lumberjacks, and this undoubtedly explains why athletes are less subject to appendicitis. Anyhow, it is quite evident that we have lost the real need for the appendix. Man at one time was supplied with an antiseptic saliva like most animals, and no doubt you have often wondered when you saw a dog or a cat eating putrid meat why the animal did not become poisoned. As the animal devours the flesh this saliva continues to pour out over the meat, which destroys the bacilli. A horse or cow does not have this natural germicide in the same degree that many other animals do, but they are supplied with a sense that does not allow them to touch unclean things, and so the horse and the cow are called clean animals. Man has entirely lost the antiseptic saliva and has retained the intuitive sense in a minor form, mostly relying upon his sight, taste and mental deduction to save him from being poisoned. But for all this the vital sources remain the same in a man now, as they did a hundred thousand years ago. If anything, perhaps they are intensified. Offhand you might say that our vital sources lie within our nervous system, the heart, lungs, liver and kidneys. Quite true, but there are a lot of other vital aids in which I believe you would be interested.

Here is an amusing incident that will make you smile, but it opens up a debatable point, and in the end proves the value of physical exercise. I was visiting a friend, and on the lawn some children were playing. One had run so much that he was all out of breath and ran over to an older child to rest on the ground, where he lay panting for breath. The older child chided the other with childish philosophy for running so much. After a little while the younger child looked up at his companion and asked, "If I breathe more slowly will I live longer?" You smile, but at the same time if you see a runner training you are apt to advise him to stop breathing through his mouth. Your advice is as wrong as the question of the child. Nature has a way of taking care of our breathing, deciding whether it should be fast or slow, through the mouth or not. Right at the base of the brain is a nerve center which is extremely sensitive to the amount of carbon dioxide that is in the blood. If there is more carbon dioxide than what there should be in the blood, the nerve center responds to the occasion by sending out nerve messages to the muscles of the chest that will quicken the rise and fall of the chest, so that you will breathe more rapidly, drawing the fresh air into the lungs. Now you know that running requires more energy and requires the living cells, mainly in the muscles, to work faster in order to throw off carbon dioxide which therefore becomes in excess the amount which the lungs can properly take care of. This makes the nerve center in your brain become alarmed, and compels you to breathe faster and faster until you finally pant. In order to pant you must open your mouth, which when done under extreme exertion like running or climbing up a long flight of stairs is a natural method of recuperation by expelling carbon dioxide as the oxygen is inhaled. The great value of exercise is that it rids the body of the fatigue toxins that clog the living tissues of the muscles and secrete within the cells. This is all caught up in the blood stream, and then discharged from the body.

Speaking about running, climbing and the attendant exertion, gives us another lesson in gravity, and the reason why nature has equipped us with larger muscles in the legs than the arms, or anywhere else for that matter. When you go up a hill you are actually lifting your weight against the force of gravity. It may surprise you to know that if you weigh one hundred and fifty pounds and you run up a hill in one minute, far enough so that you rise a vertical distance of ten feet, you are using the power equivalent to one twentieth of a horse power to thus handle your one hundred and fifty pounds bodyweight. This takes muscular power to transport you and oxygen for fuel. You can readily see that if your body is out of condition, you have a real task ahead of you in merely handling yourself.

If people would only stop for a few minutes to think of the great necessity of keeping fit, there would not be a person in the country who would not be taking exercise in one form or another. If everybody could realize how much one part of the body must help the other, even just by stimulating the circulation of the blood stream and keeping it free of impurities, they would relieve certain organisms of much unnecessary work, and thus preserve them for other emergencies. Did you ever consider when you cut your hand how it was that you were saved from infection? In the blood stream are millions of tiny granules of whitish jelly, which are white corpuscles. In reality they are the defenders of your body. Their duty is to fight and absorb all foreign substances, which seek to enter the body. When you cut yourself, they rush in great numbers to the wound and ward off any invading germs. These little men of war have a strange method of existence. They live on their prey. If a germ gets in the body they soon find it and engulf the germ inside their own body, where it apparently becomes digested. It is further claimed that there are no white corpuscles in a body that has died of sickness. Apparently they finally are absorbed in fighting disease. Really the body is the most absorbing study in existence. Nothing is so intricate, perplexing or so wonderful, yet it is claimed that the ingredients that constitute a one hundred and fifty pound body have only a market value of ninety-eight cents. Well, figure it out, just for the interest it will afford you. About two-thirds of the total weight is water. I have seen it estimated that the average one hundred and fifty pound body contains ten gallons of water, about twenty-four pounds of carbon and seven pounds of lime, then there are two ounces of phosphorus and a little less than two ounces of salt. About one quarter of iron, one-fifth of sugar, and very small amounts of potassium, sculpture, magnesium, fluorine and iodine. Nearly five pounds of nitrogen, and thirteen pounds of hydrogen and oxygen, in addition to what is contained in water. Nearly all the chemical changes in our body take place within a solution of water. Sometimes, when too much salt gets into the blood, we are obliged to drink a considerable quantity of water in order to wash it away. Thirst is always a sign that the body needs more water for such purposes.

"Let nature take its course" is an old adage that wears well. Dame nature never makes a mistake. We generally make them instead. I like to study nature as it really takes its course, and have often found a great deal of interest in noting certain similar likes in people of all nations. The liking for sweet things seemed to have always existed. In the history of barbaric nations mention is made of the use of sweet meats. At one time I had the impression that the taste for all things that contained sugar was more or less a civilized innovation; but I have found the liking for sugar to be universal with all beings that live out of water. A bear loves honey, a horse likes sugar, and a cow, sweet clover; and where sugar is not obtainable among savage races sweet juices and foods were used as a substitute. I began to realize that sugar played a very important part in the existence of certain physical changes. Now we know it is so. The muscles cannot do without it. The main function of the liver is to conserve and control the amount of sugar that is distributed in the blood. When you eat sugar it is absorbed and carried to the liver. There the liver converts it into a substance called glycogen, and as the muscles require more sugar, the liver converts a little of this glycogen back into sugar and releases it into the blood stream so that it can be carried to the muscles that require it. This will give you a little idea of what is meant by that old question when one asks another, "How's your liver?" If that is all right, you are generally all right.

Another of our ancestral aversions peculiar to all mankind, is the natural dislike of anything very sour. These two traits have not been sacrificed in evolution. Much as the sense of a horse forbids it to touch unclean food by scent, man once relied entirely upon taste to determine good food from bad. If it was sour, it was thrown away, as sour foods contain acids, which are often dangerous. Maybe the term "horse sense" is an ancient tribute to this ability to know right from wrong.

Nature has a way of protecting us if we are only willing to heed her. Give her a chance to serve you and you will be better off for it. So many ask me just how often they should exercise and how many repetitions they should practice in any exercise; and many will say that although they get very tired when exercising, yet they plug away. I do not approve of anything like that. When a pupil starts in training it is quite possible to schedule the number of repetitions for each exercise over a period of a few months. But when his progress becomes so advanced that heavier poundages are required, the going is not so easy. Then he has to use judgment. He can always be told approximately what he should do, but no day is ever exactly like another. A mental worry, heavier daily work than usual, a meal that did not exactly agree with you, any one of a number of things is likely to happen which will leave more fatigue toxins in the system than is ordinarily the case, or a depression is felt upon the blood stream. In the end, one of these little annoyances has deprived us of a little more energy than usual, and exercise becomes a little harder that night. There is no use in being excited over a little thing like that. Cater to it, for it is nature that is asserting itself. Be satisfied to do a little less. It will help you more, and when you are feeling extra peppy, train that much harder. Many are worried by the fact that on Thursday night they did not have the same pep that they had on Tuesday. Why if they did, every athlete would always be at top form, and the thrill would be taken out of competition. It is this uncertainty that makes life and sport a gamble. But the man who knows his body best, with its little peculiarities, will always go further in both body building and playing games.

I remember a young boxer who was showing some extraordinary talent, but he was always afraid of his mid-section. The only time he had been counted out was from a punch to the solar plexus. Twice he had met the canvas from such blows. He told me that he must have an unusual weakness there, which in the end would rob him of his chance to succeed. I reasoned with him along these lines. "Look here, how many knockouts are registered as the result of a solar plexus blow? About one out of ten. The reason this happens is that fighters intuitively go for the jaw. Few concentrate upon the solar plexus as their target. Now, if you had lost both of those bouts by a slam on the jaw you would have thought less about it, because you have been taught to believe that no matter how strong or good a boxer is, a blow on the point of the jaw will put him out. This being true, it is more true that a blow to the solar plexus, while not making a man unconscious, will make him just as helpless, and he will suffer more for this reason. At the pit of the stomach is a little knot of important nerves that are very sensitive. A blow over that mark will upset the whole nervous organism. It can happen to any man. Now as this is a nervous condition, your mind will affect it. If you keep thinking about it, your brain is continually sending out its nerve waves to the solar plexus center to beware, which in turn excites these nerves and makes them more sensitive. It is different with the knockout on the jaw. There is a little vein that runs up the side of the jaw to the brain, and when a man is struck on the point of the jaw the jaw is knocked sideways, and momentarily stops the flow of blood from this vein to the brain, which causes a momentary concussion that puts you out until circulation becomes normal. So you see, both blows will put any one out." I advised him not to worry about it, and just build the muscles of protection to as nearly prefect a state as possible and he would have less cause to worry about his solar plexus than his jaw. He told me later that the explanation was worth a thousand dollars to him, as it showed him that he was not the victim of an unusual weakness. Anyhow, he never suffered another such knockout and climbed high in the boxing game.

Nature will give you an answer to most of your questions, if you are willing to study, but never make the fatal mistake of bucking nature. She will not stand for it. I can safely say that in all my studies of the body and its mechanisms I always take into consideration what nature had first ordained that certain part to do. This fixed in mind and clearly understood, I am better able to map out a plan. I have never advocated anything that I did not do myself, and I never advocate methods as being acceptable to the other man, when I know the method is only permissible to one or two people by reason of a peculiar physical construction that the given person may possess. You can find a way if you study yourself. Nature is an open book for all those who will leaf the pages. She is not secretive, but above board rather than anything else. Allowances are made for everything, for natural compensation is more just and exact than the best insurance company in the world. You cannot fool nature. She will make you pay someday, but you can help her by keeping yourself fit. Nature thrives on exercise. So, by exercise we are able to build better bodies than those possessed by our forbears. It is foolish to say that the ancients were healthier than we are, or that they were free from disease. We are all born of the flesh, and we must all die, and death only comes from accident, sickness and old age. King Tutankhamen died of tuberculosis and the Pharaoh that led the Israelites into captivity died of cancer. There are a multitude of vital spots in the body, only a few on which I have touched, but like your heart, lungs, liver and kidneys, they must all be considered in your study and practice of body culture. Of course, you do not have to study each one separately, that would be almost impossible. What I have written here gives you a little idea of what goes on within yourself and what you possess. When any of these vital spots go wrong, we suffer, and the cause is invariably traceable to lack of body toning or faulty organic or muscular construction brought about by neglect. All you have to do is to condition your body and all these other factors will become benefited in turn. It all ends up with physical training. I hope you will find this little talk interesting enough to lead you into the paths of observation and study to find out more for yourself, and profit more from the value of intensive body building.

CHAPTER XXIII
THE STANDARD THAT DETERMINES THE IDEAL SHAPE

There is no doubt in my mind that Eugene Sandow's rise to fame was due more to the symmetrical shapeliness of his enviable body than to the difficulty of feats of strength he performed. Generally speaking, there are two things which will always impress the mind of the body culturist, shape and strength. With strength, we have already dealt. Therefore, we will now direct our attention to the value of shapeliness, and the influence it has upon our mind and body. Oh yes, it has a great influence upon the mind. The next time you visit an art gallery notice the quiet reverence that is displayed by the art lovers, as they move from one picture to another. The serene beauty of the pictures permeates the whole atmosphere, leaving the beholders in silent wonder. I have a great friend who is a wonderful artist, and he often makes sketches of the body in varied postures, which he brings to me for my scrutiny. On one of his visits he said to me, "I can always tell whether the drawings meet with your approval or not. Not by what you say, as much as by how little you say. Your eyes are always drawn to the pictures you like best, and I have noticed that you have sometimes been so enraptured that you did not hear me speak to you." He was quite right. Pictures of the body beautiful, correctly translated, never weary me. I can feast my eyes upon them for hours at a time. This rather contradicts the statement that, familiarity with the most beautiful objects, breeds contempt. For twenty-five years I have lived in the atmosphere of beautiful bodies, and I am still as enthusiastic as I was when I first commenced my studies.

Universally the young body builder will accept for his ideal the athlete whose form is symmetrically formed, in preference to the man who is known for his great strength alone. If an athlete is so fortunate as to possess both these attributes, he is idolized even more. I believe it was this exceptional combination possessed by George Hackenschmidt that made him my lifelong ideal. We all have our ideal. Just as the athlete of today accepted Sandow, Hackenschmidt and others, as their inspiration in their early days, so is the young body idealist of to-day inspired by the magnificent body of men like Adolph Nordquest, Staff Sergeant Moss and Siegmund Klein among others. Each is striving to mould the shape of his body on the same lines of his ideal, and each will in turn become the example for the generation of body builders of tomorrow.

About the first thing a body builder does is to inquire about the measurements of his ideal along with his other habits. Irrespective of his own weight and structure, he jumps into his training with the idea that some day he is going to have the same muscular dimensions. In other words, he struggles to imitate and duplicate in every way. He is all wrong there. If he had to concentrate on securing the same proportions, according to his height as his ideal, he would then be on the right track.

Measurements have become almost a curse in determining what the ideal figure should be. No two men are built alike, even though they are the same height and bodyweight. If one man has larger feet and hands, or if his head is larger than another, his appearance will be very different. His hips may be large, or the clavicles of his shoulders may be short, in either of which case he will have to change his ideas on his own ideal measurements. The condition of these two parts will influence your whole build, as much as the size of the hands, feet and head. As I said in a previous chapter, do not bother about your boney structure in determining the proportions you should acquire in order to achieve the ideal physical state. Let your height guide you first, then see how the rest of your body measures up. If your hips are large, the thighs are likely to be heavy, and if your hands are large, your forearm is likely to be larger in proportion than your biceps. All these points have to be taken into consideration first, and then you have to lay out a routine that will satisfactorily bring up the smaller parts to balance with the heavier parts.

Where shapeliness is the supreme desire, care will have to be taken to see that all the muscles are balanced and shaped. Your measurements are not going to tell you this. Your upper arm may span sixteen inches, but that does not mean to say the triceps will balance with the biceps. The same thing applies to the legs. As a rule the biceps of the thigh is below par, and the absence of that muscle certainly takes away from the beauty of the thigh formation. Balance. That word is the key to a beautiful physique. It is your balanced appearance when stripped that will always decide the issue before judges, and not primarily what your measurements are. As the body becomes balanced the measurements will be taken care of in their own way.

The art of posing has become a very prominent one in a body culturist's program. At one time he sought only to excel at tumbling, wrestling, or lifting weights, and when he stripped for a picture he would generally strike some pose in which his muscles bulged into horrible postures that made him appear to be a grotesque being. This has passed away, and the poseur's art has developed a better understanding of the body. Today we are capable of displaying the body in graceful, flowing lines that clearly enhance the value of body building, and do not detract from the suggestion of strength.

At one time the Apollo style was greatly in vogue, and many sought to duplicate these effeminate lines; but this example never had general favor, for nature calls for a man to look like a man, and not like an undeveloped girl. The Theseus form was discovered and found to fill the need of a masculine ideal more satisfactorily. This is now the accepted standard as it was in the ages past, when that statue was first made. It combines the graces of Apollo and the sturdy strength of a normalized Hercules. I have often studied the statues of the Apollo Belvedere, and the Farnese Hercules, and I could only see one quality in either, neither seemed to have the proper combination. The Apollo suggested grace, poise and beauty, but the form was too feminine to be perfect. It bespoke under development more than anything else, for the legs are heavy in proportion to the slim, straight lines of the upper body. The Farnese Hercules is just as badly exaggerated the other way, and the legs are way out of proportion also. Just the same, the suggestion is there, making us realize its colossal power. In Praxtiles, Theseus, we find the most appealing form. It breathes power, manly beauty and gracefulness. There is no standard of measurement to actually determine how you can know whether you have the Theseus form or not. You simply cultivate your muscles so that they will balance.

One day my artist friend and I were talking this subject over, and during the discussion I took out a number of photographic poses of several well known body culturists, including Hackenschmidt, Staff Sergeant Moss, Dandurand, Bobby Pandour, Chas. MacMahon and Siegmund Klein. Spreading these out on my desk, I asked my friend to pick out the most perfect type of manhood. He couldn't. Every man drew his admiration. Finally he remarked, "There is no choice among them. They are all wonderful." He was surprised when I told him that their body- weights ranged from one hundred and forty-seven pounds to two hundred and ten pounds, which goes to prove that no matter how tall, or how short you are, the Theseus standard can be applied to all. Study their attitude in every pose. There is nothing forced in their positions. They are wonderfully natural. Some of the measurements of some of these men would not impress you at all, as against the measurements of Hackenschmidt, which again goes to prove my statement that balance rather than measurements is what counts. Every muscle is shaped, rounded or curved in the most exquisite lines. For instance, take the legs of Moss and MacMahon; I don't care from what position you view them, they are a glorious interpretation of muscular anatomy. Balanced with the hips and calves, they explain to you much better than I can write, how a pair of legs should look. Incidentally both of these men are artists' models of international reputation. Charles MacMahon has done more posing than any other model I know of in this country. His services are always in great demand. He led the movement away from the effeminate poses characterized by those who were led to believe that the Apollo Belvedere was the correct form. All his casts like those of Moss and Hackenschmidt depict life, vigor or rest, according to the study. The Greeks never produced any more beautiful specimen in their physical entirety. Klein and Pandour, both have torsos of such magnificent formation that they will live like the glories of Greece, always. Hackenschmidt and Dandurand are men of weight, and vital types who radiate power in every symmetrical line and curve of their body. I have known all of these poseurs personally. I know how their adamite bodies strike the eye and impress the mind when you see them pose. The magnetic influence they radiate compels you to become a body culturist without a mention of the fact. However, their qualities do not begin and end merely as expositors of the body, as each man is possessed of the extraordinary speed, suppleness and strength that makes them efficient athletes.

You will notice in the physiques of each of these men, a very fine tapering off of the body. Commencing with the breadth of the shoulders, a slope begins that gives the body a well balanced V shape as it finishes at the feet. The neck should be a little larger than the biceps, about an inch, and

313

the calf should be about a half inch to three quarters smaller than the biceps. There are all kinds of measurement tables on the market, but none of them have stood the test of time. Some of them are utterly ridiculous. From the mass of information that I have collected over the years on measurements, I made an average of the measurements as they are possessed by the majority of the best built and strongest men in each class. These measurements I am including because I know the interest among all body builders for such. You will find them quite different to most you have seen, but these are the actual measurements of the majority per height that really looked more like what we are after. These measurements, as you see, are made up with a gap of two inches between each tabulation because I find that five feet four inches and five feet five inches and so on have too much similarity to consider, and they also cover the ages from eighteen years up.

	Weight	Neck	Chest	Waist	Biceps	Forearms	Wrist	Hips	Thighs	Calf
5'4"	145	15½	39	29	14½	12	7	33	22	14
5'6"	160	16	41	31	15	12¼	7¾	34	23	14½
5'8"	175	16½	43	32	16	13	7½	36	23½	15
5'10"	190	17½	45	33	16½	13½	7¾	38	24	16
6'	200	18	47	35	17	13½	8	39	25½	16½

I want to draw your attention to a few facts as I see them. You will notice that the five foot four and five foot six inch grades, have larger waists by comparison with the chest on the average, than the men in the five feet ten inches and six foot grades. This is due to their more compact bodies, which has less space between the ribs and the hips. For the opposite reason have the five feet ten inch and six feet grades apparently got a more trim waist. That is, their waist covers a greater length and the mass of tissue is naturally distributed over a longer area. The five foot eight inch

314

grade jumps an inch in waist difference, making a difference of eleven inches between chest and Waist as against ten inches in the first two grades and twelve inches in the last two, but you will find his extra weight is accounted for by a bigger jump in biceps and calf size than any of the others, and his hip measurement jumps higher by two inches over the five feet six inch grade. It is in this grade that we find men of great vitality. These few facts will prove to you the unreliability of measurements in determining what proportions a man should have in order to build for himself the ideal shape. Take Hackenschmidt for example, he stood less than six feet and stripped at two hundred and ten pounds, his measurements are way above the six foot grade, but no one can find a fault with that masterpiece. Charles MacMahon stands about five feet eight inches and weighs one hundred and eighty pounds, his measurements run a little better than the five foot eight inch grade but anyone would be proud to own a physique like his. If you want to accept measurements according to statistics, then you can safely accept these tables as being somewhat approximate, but you will be obliged to consider your physical peculiarities in order to be more definite. When I see a man I can tell right away pretty near how he should shape up, as I immediately take into consideration the points that I have explained in this chapter. But you will find it just to be as I have stated, that it is entirely your appearance as you strip that will count the most of all in acquiring the shape which is best described as "Sculptor Form."

CHAPTER XXIV
SOME ACTUAL RESULTS OF PRACTICAL EXERCISE

The quality of a system is always judged by the results that it has achieved, not so much in one or two isolated cases through a brief trial as over a period of time among a great number. The actual results in exercise are more important than the actual results in business, as judged by the fact that as long as you have health and strength you can recuperate from a business reverse, but when the body is badly impaired, the value of life and its achievements are both lost. Money cannot buy health and strength. Nature sets too high a value on these gifts and will not barter them for gold. In this she is worse than a Shylock, exacting her due to the last fraction, even if it has to be your life that is forfeited. However, to those who are willing to follow her promptings, she is wonderfully generous and bountiful. During my lifetime, I have watched thousands upon thousands of health seekers take up the reins of right living, and have seen the actual results achieved. Many have actually passed through my hands, and I am glad to know that I have helped to a certain extent, to place this glorious gospel of body culture in many places. It has a fascination for me, and I am justly proud of some of the products whose wonderful bodies and glorious achievements were the results of my efforts. Some of these examples I am going to bring before you, and show you in just what condition they were when they took up this great work, and I hope that the lesson their life provides will make some of you ashamed of yourselves, and all of you determined to go and do better.

My first example is going to be of one young man, who, while entirely unknown to any of my readers, or the athletic world, became one of my cherished friends. It all happened like this. Some years ago I was standing in the doorway of my shop, after having taken an invigorating workout in the gymnasium that was on the floor above. I was happy and enjoying the fullness of good health. I always seemed to feel a greater gratitude and exhilaration as I felt the blood coursing quickly through my veins, and the muscles smoothly gliding under my skin after a workout. One of those "God is Good" feelings. Approaching me, from the left side of the street, was a slim, young fellow, about five feet seven inches tall. He aroused my curiosity as I noticed he was not whistling. I did not know much about him, but whether I was inside the shop or not I could always tell if he were passing because he was always whistling. Of course, he had the privilege of not whistling for once if he liked and I suppose you might figure he was entitled to a rest once in a while. That was not it. When you know a chap to have a definite habit, and to be always laughing or whistling, every hour of the day, there is something psychologically wrong when he makes an omission. Human nature does not work that way. The nearer he came the more my belief that something was wrong was confirmed. His eyes were fixed on the pavement, and a look of abject misery was pictured upon his face. His stride seemed to wilt under the serious oppression of his thoughts. Mental telepathy, if you want to call it such, signaled to me, and for the first time I spoke to him. He did not hear me; but I spoke again, asking him how he was. His face twitched as he mumbled a reply and his step faltered. I felt an awful pity for him, as I could plainly see that he was sick. I drew him inside and invited him to tell me what was wrong. It was a story that has been told before, but he was one of the exceptions, who was reaping the harvest of his wild oats too early in life. He had always had weak lungs and a combination of the violent dissipation of youth and neglect had set their seal upon him. Tuberculosis. He had just come from the doctor, who had

317

ordered him not to work for one year. The mountains and a sanatorium were prescribed, as usual, but the boy had no money and he had a home to help support. I talked to him for over an hour, and told him I was sure I could help him if he would do as I told him. It was the straw to the drowning man's clutch, and he tearfully grabbed it. I got him just in time. Within two weeks he was sleeping restfully, without the torture of the racking cough. A month, and he was a changed being. Six weeks, and he was back doing light work, and inside of three months he was working in the factory at his former job. He trained and followed instructions as only one who is fighting for his life will. During that time I had kept him with me all the time. If I had occasion to drive out of town he went with me, although we were totally unlike in our make-ups and I was easily ten years older than he. But as he found that his strength was returning and he was actually getting better than he had ever been in his life, the pall of my more serious nature began to bore him. Gradually he slipped back into the old life, and I seldom saw him. I had done all I had promised, and it was his own life he was living, so I figured it was useless to say anything to him, for he was old enough to know better. Despite our opposite nature I had grown to like this nineteen-year-old boy. Whenever I did see him he was the same laughing, merry, whistling boy, who had already developed an affection towards me. A year slid by and with it a tale was retold. There are some things with which a man can be fooled, but no one can hide certain conditions from one who has spent his life doing one thing. Whenever I saw Don I noticed the gradual sinking of the cheeks, and the shadows that were forming under the eyes, and that little hacking cough which he began to blame on cigarettes. But he began to avoid me, and I had no intention of going out of my way to play the good Samaritan if my aid was not required. One evening his sister called on me and told me everything. He was

318

ashamed to come back after he had realized his folly. The upshot was that he came back, but the struggle was much harder this time. I had told him that I could not promise anything a second time, but he had to choose between the straight and narrow path, once and for all, or disaster. He was a game fighter, and he made good. Better still, he remained good. From a horrible wreck of about one hundred pounds, he built up into as tough a piece of man flesh at one hundred and fifty pounds as I ever saw. He would wrestle with me like a demon as one of my partners, and he played on the forward line of the football team I captained. We developed an inseparable friendship, with absolute devotion on his part. He had learned his lesson and swallowed his medicine like a man, fully realizing the value of it and what exercise could do for him. He is settled down now, with a fine little wife and a child to bless their home. We were nearer than brothers. He never left my side, and was always the last to grasp my hand as I stepped into the arena and the first when I stepped out. My honor was his honor, for which he would fight like a tiger. I helped him back to health, and gained one of the finest pals a man ever had, which balanced the scales perfectly.

I am sorry if I have allowed my affection for a friend to lead me to digress from the actual subject, but still this example proves what can be obtained from a clean life built up from following the true principle of body culture. Also the story of Frank Dennis affords one of the finest instances of how low a man can be pulled down, and how high he can rise. Dennis was a victim of the great "Flu" epidemic that swept through the country a few years ago. He developed double pneumonia, which left him with a weak heart and badly weakened lungs. He developed hemorrhages and in four days lost sixteen pounds. Invalided home from the hospital, he was a complete wreck. During his convalescence the study of body culture began to appeal to him as a means of reclaiming his lost health. At that time I was located in Pittsburgh, but he came to me, and I am very proud to say that within two years he was the winner of the middleweight weight-lifting championship of America. Actually six months after he had commenced under my supervision he had stepped into the record creating class, making his first record with a performance in the wrestler's bridge lift. From one victory he passed to another, until he secured the champion crown. His wonderfully formed body has since been an inspiration to thousands. Every line and every curve shows up with rugged strength. His chest, which was once so badly sunken, swells out in a magnificent roll, with a depth that proves the great volume of lung power that has since been his. There has not been the slightest recurrence of either heart or lung affection since he started rebuilding his wasted frame. To look at his hefty pair of legs no one would believe he ever had such a thing as a weak heart, for the legs are the hardest members of the body to build up when such has been the trouble. Care and patience must be always remembered, otherwise the great quantity of blood that is required to nourish these big leg muscles would keep the heart in a weakened state. Dennis is like most people who have come up from the shadow of the grave. He is a zealous apostle of body building, and never loses an opportunity to demonstrate his vast physical capabilities for the benefit of others. The occasion when Dennis laid down and allowed an automobile to run over his abdomen is fitting evidence of the quality of his muscular resistance. He had no cushions under him as a protection, neither did he have sloping blocks for the car to run up on and off, like other performers. He simply laid on the road and allowed the machine to run over him in order to prove an argument.

Then we have the case of Charles Shaffer, another star athlete, who has graced the vaudeville stage with his impressive physique and super-athletic abilities. Shaffer is only a small man, but he is a veritable dynamo of energy.

Struck down with double pneumonia, he almost left this world behind him, and his convalescence was so slow that all hope was abandoned on several occasions. However, the spark of life lingered and grew, and as soon as he was out of bed he began to make plans for the future. I had the great pleasure of taking him in hand and guiding him until he went on the stage. He advanced more rapidly than any other man I ever knew. As his body began to develop he formed a great inclination for hand-balancing and tumbling. It was a step I greatly encouraged, although he made his athletic debut as a wrestler on the Pittsburgh "Y" wrestling team, and cleaned up honors in two classes in one night. In his advanced stages of training he took up the sport of weight lifting, and made some remarkable records that still stand. The unusual development of his body began to excite attention, and he took up the art of posing. With all credit due to all of the splendidly built athletes I know, I believe that Shaffer has the most outstanding muscular development of any. Every muscle stands out as clearly separated from the other as though each one was chiseled out of marble, and he has remarkable control over them all. He succeeded John Fielding as the bantamweight weight-lifting champion of America. Fielding was another of the many who had come under my tutelage and climbed to the top. He came under my direction when he was in his thirties, after he had tried the best specialists in Europe, Britain and this country to overcome an organic trouble. I was, fortunately, successful with this Massachusetts athlete, who became known as the "Pocket Hercules." Fielding retired from active competition with honors, but with all due respects to my earlier protégé, I have to say that Shaffer was the daddy of them all in his bodyweight class. He is a Hercules in miniature, overshadowing for both strength and physical development such stars as Artie Edmunds, Paolo, and Luis Hardt, also ranking as one of the greatest hand-balancing performers that ever stepped on the

321

vaudeville stage. He became so interested in the demonstration of physical efficiency that he forsook a lucrative occupation to become a professional performer. While remarking about the skillful abilities of Shaffer, and the former pupils, it came to my mind that some readers may wonder why I include these facts, as it can be easily recognized that I do not mention their feats solely as a proof of how good they became. You will notice that they became adept in a certain line of sport quite early in their body building process. It really was a part of their program. I always studied their athletic inclinations. Whether they had any previous athletic ability before taking up body culture or not, their interest quickly developed in one certain sport. I fostered this interest, for I always found it a very valuable aid. It increased their enthusiasm, and they could see the actual results of their labors as they went along.

At the time of the disbanding of the troops after the war, one young man, who was the son of a local minister, had broken down under the rigors of the Russian front. He was discharged as medically unfit, developing lung trouble from exposure and pneumonia. He was a sorry looking sight when his father brought him to me. Standing about six feet three inches, he weighed about one hundred and twenty pounds, and his whole appearance was one of emaciation. However, he built up rapidly, and I got him interested in fencing. He became quite adept at the foil game, and within six months of starting training, dating from the night of his introduction to me, he was representing his university in the national fencing tournament. He won second place, losing by just one point. I have not seen him for a few years, but I do not have to see him. He has been shown what has to be done, and he got the full benefits of the results. I know he has brains enough never to forget the value of the teachings of exercise, and so I know that he still keeps up a valuable policy.

All who come to my attention are not, by any means, the victims of ill health, but rarely has one come forward who had plainly evidenced the great possibilities that he finally developed. Take Marineau and Fournier for instance. They both were very ordinary young men in the first place. Any other ordinary person of their weight could equal them, but they took a great interest in the study of body building and finally became keen adherents to the sport of weight lifting. Their success and great achievements in that sport are due to diligence, perseverance and an intelligent application of right training principles.

I remember when I was training on the other side, a man of about thirty-eight years of age came to see me at my training quarters. He was a Sandow pupil and a very wealthy English business man. Indigestion had been the bane of his life for years, and all medical help seemed futile. He became a pupil of Sandow at the suggestion of another athlete with whom I was acquainted at that time. Sandow certainly made a man of him, but it is the other fellow I want to tell you about. His name was George Heywood. He was the son of a millionaire English manufacturer, and when I knew him he was a fine specimen of manhood, and a crack amateur bike rider of those days. Bronchitis and heart trouble had cost his father a small fortune, and finally his despairing parents were told that it was useless to go further. His son might live six months, but nine months was hardly possible. Quiet and rest were advised, and an army of attendants waited on his every move and call. One day George put the proposition up to his father like this, "Listen, dad, you have done all you can for me, and we have tried everything but one thing, and I want you to let me try it. There is no use of your kicking, for I am going to die anyway, and I much prefer dying trying to get health, rather than waiting for death to claim me." The son got his own way, and Sandow was responsible for his cure. What amazed me the most was, that in less than six months afterwards he competed in a one hundred mile bike race and won it. Of all sports bike racing makes the heart work harder than any other. Heywood was a splendid wrestler, gymnast and weight lifter, and I used to enjoy seeing him work out. When we wrestled he would bore in like a young lion, and the sparkle in his snapping eyes shot out glimpses of the buoyant energy and joy of living that he was enjoying.

A very interesting case arose in connection with one of my clients. He was twenty-nine years of age and had never been able to raise his right hand to his head since he was a boy. He got started and about three months afterwards he was happily showing me that he could comb his hair with that hand, put on his hat, and almost straighten his arm overhead, which he ultimately did.

I have had the pleasure of handling a great number of men, with great success, who lost the use of certain muscles as a result of injury in the World War; but there are no miracles about such cures if you want to call them that. They are much as I wrote in the chapter on "Curative Exercise." The physician had done his work and the rest was left to exercise. It is just a logical application of the right method of physical training. Remedial gymnastics was a godsend to the gassed, paralyzed, and semi-paralyzed soldiers of the World War. When all medical aid had been given the patients were turned over to the training corps who understood this special work. The statistics showed that eighty- seven and a half per cent, of the patients were returned to civilian life, cured and one hundred per cent fit. Is that not wonderful? Try to realize that if it had not been for remedial gymnastics all those men would have been thrown back into the wage-earning struggle, handicapped, incompetent to hold down their former jobs. There are thousands upon thousands of disabled soldiers who have a heart full of praise for the value of exercise.

Of recent years one of my best productions is Albert Manger, the well known Baltimore weight lifter. Manger, within eighteen months, developed from a sickly, under developed man of one hundred and twenty-nine pounds to one hundred and eighty-two pounds of as fine a piece of manhood as you would wish to see. The moment he strips he arrests the eyes. To look at him you would imagine he weighed two hundred pounds, so massive are his muscular proportions, and his ability to lift in both slow and fast lifts bears witness to the splendid co-ordination of speed and strength that he possesses, Then there is David P. Willoughby, the famous Pacific Coast athlete, who, while only a light heavyweight, won the American heavyweight weight-lifting championship. He was formerly a slender, almost scrawny, individual when he first took up progressive training, and I can safely say that at the present time he is one of the finest athletes. He started out training as a much under developed young man and developed into a world's champion in his bodyweight class. Coulter is remarkable in many ways. He is one of the few of the great athletes who allowed his studies to take him to a real depth below the surface, which is all so many bother with. I have a great admiration for him as a man and an athlete, and he has been a great help in promoting the cause of right thinking, with right exercise, in this country. He has a marvelous control over his body, and I believe he was the pioneer introducing muscle control in America.

When Siegmund Klein took up progressive body training he was only a very ordinarily built young man, but most of you are familiar with the splendid results he obtained for himself. As I allow my mind to consider some of the obstacles with which many body builders have had to contend, I am inclined to become provoked at others. The truth is, that many young fellows do not know how well off they are when they start in. Just think of the struggle Joe Nordquest had. He lost his leg below the knee in an accident, when he was a young boy; this set him back considerably. Originally he did not have a husky foundation to start with, as many imagine. He was quite light, and there were times when he began to think that he would never succeed, but Adolph, his elder brother, and one of the most magnificent athletes America ever developed, was always a source of inspiration to him. With that one great handicap he continued to plug away, and it took time to get there, but he got there just the same. He practiced weight lifting and became extraordinarily efficient in all forms of strength, and has raised enormous poundages in various lifts. Although Joe has retired from the sport, yet his name, his feats and his powerful physique will retain an honored place in the history of the strong man and muscle builder in this country. Despite his great weight he became a fine hand balancer, and was the heaviest man I ever knew who could make a single hand stand. Another incident that claimed my admiration, in which an athlete was handicapped with the loss of a limb, was Charles Maw, an English boy. He weighed about one hundred and twenty-six pounds. As the result of an accident his arm was taken completely off, but this plucky little man went into the field of muscle culture with a bang. He acquired a wonderful body, and in the bent press he was credited with a lift of two hundred and twenty-four pounds.

One incident brings to mind another. Anyhow, I was very familiar with an officer who had served overseas and lost his leg, and was distracted to know what he would do when he returned to civilian life. By profession he was a surveyor, and naturally his casualty eliminated him from that occupation. I knew he was a good jumper, so I suggested to him to take up training again, built his body up, and study balancing to control equipoise. He did, and made such a success of it that he became a professional performer, and made a better and easier living than he had in pre-war days.

H. E. Keeseckin, of Peoria, Illinois, was discharged from the Marine Corps for heart trouble. He later came under my attention and within eighteen months he wrought a marvelous change in himself. Organically and physically he became perfect, as did A. Batsis, who was such a wreck from stomach and intestinal disorder, that he only weighed about ninety pounds at the start of his training. Nine months later he displayed a body that was a real prize winner, and I had the pleasure of making him over.

These are just a few of the men, out of thousands, who got practical results from following practical body building exercise. I have not picked only the best examples, for I know of others who have become greater even than Nordquest. There were men who had to fight the ravages of lung trouble, liver and kidney disorders, heart weakness and the disadvantage of crippled limbs, like O. Martin, of Attica, Indiana, who suffered with infantile paralysis, and today is one of our shining examples of physical fitness. What they all had to encounter and overcome, and the final achievements they secured in build and ability, should be a real inspirational lesson to everyone who does not have any of these things with which to contend. To those who have, these examples should be a beacon to guide them to the greatest goal that life presents. The value of their success cannot be judged in gold or priceless jewels. In itself, it is the incomparable prize, a glorified body, that is fighting fit with health and strength, obtained by the handiwork of nature through its servant, progressive body culture.

Made in the USA
Lexington, KY
14 February 2015